THE GOOD DOCTOR

In this engaging, authoritative and compassionate book, Paterson draws on decades of experience in public service to pose and answer four questions: what is the ideal 'good doctor'? What is the reality of medical practice – including the problem of the 'poorly performing practitioner' – in New Zealand and other nations with comparable health care systems? What are the barriers to moving medical practice closer to the ideal? And what can we improve, using the legal, regulatory and other tools on hand? Demonstrating a deep knowledge of how health care really works, respect for the challenges faced by patients and physicians alike and a deft use of case studies to illustrate problems and opportunities for improvement, Paterson aims to 'prompt debate and lead to change'. This book should be essential reading for medical professionals and health care policy-makers in New Zealand, and is likely of be of great interest to patients and their advocates.
— NANCY BERLINGER, PHD MDIV, THE HASTINGS CENTER

Most doctors are competent and altruistic. A few are incompetent and altruistic. A few are competent but exploitative. A tiny minority are incompetent and exploitative. Good systems, good premises and political correctness do little to protect consumers. Patient satisfaction has little to do with consumer protection. Clinically incompetent doctors are also incompetent in self-assessment. Attending medical meetings does not correlate well with competence. Ron Paterson's long international experience of medical error and medical regulation has given him unique insight. His solution – proper recertification based on enhanced competence checks and remedial education focused on identified shortcomings – is so logical it must surely have its day. If he is judged to be right, as he should be, then the public, the press, the politicians and the profession must work together toward that end.
— IAN ST GEORGE, MD FRACP FRNZCGP DIPED

THE GOOD DOCTOR

WHAT PATIENTS WANT

RON PATERSON

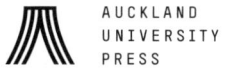

AUCKLAND
UNIVERSITY
PRESS

First published 2012
Reprinted 2012, 2019

Auckland University Press
University of Auckland
Private Bag 92019
Auckland 1142, New Zealand
www.press.auckland.ac.nz

© Ron Paterson, 2012

ISBN 978 1 86940 592 2

National Library of New Zealand Cataloguing-in-Publication Data
Paterson, Ron, 1955–
The good doctor : what patients want / by Ron Paterson.
Includes bibliographical references and index.
ISBN 978-1-86940-592-2
1. Physician and patient. 2. Physicians. 3. Medical care—
Quality control. I. Title.
610.696—dc 23

This book is copyright. Apart from fair dealing for the purpose of private study, research, criticism or review, as permitted under the Copyright Act, no part may be reproduced by any process without prior permission of the publisher.

Published with the kind assistance of

Cover design: Jason Gabbert
Cover image: Shutterstock.com
Printed in China by Everbest Printing Investment Ltd

for Mike and for Charlotte

CONTENTS

Preface ix

Part 1
The good doctor: the ideal 1

Part 2
Problem doctors: part of the reality 25

Part 3
The roadblocks: why is change so difficult? 61

Part 4
Prescription for change: what can we improve? 107

Epilogue 162
Acknowledgements 166
Notes 169
Select Bibliography 195
Index 198

PREFACE

The 'good doctor'. Every patient wants one. Every doctor wants to be one. It is widely accepted as a *desiratum*, something to be desired.

A lot of people have ideas about what makes a good doctor. Whenever I mentioned that I was writing this book, everyone had an opinion on what makes a good doctor, and what they expect as a patient. Many had a personal story to tell, of a good or bad doctor and being a satisfied or dissatisfied patient.

I have a collective story to tell about good doctors (and some not-so-good doctors) and patient expectations. After a decade heading New Zealand's patient complaints system – akin to an umpire between patients and doctors – I want to try to make sense of some of the powerful stories that people told our office. Some, stories of great care. But, as you would expect from a complaints-handling agency, far more tales of pain, suffering and frustration from patients and families let down by their doctor and health system. And companion stories of hurt and anger from doctors who felt like the second victim when a patient complained.

A daily diet of complaints, a watchful eye on medical scandals and inquiries in other countries (especially the United Kingdom), and exposure to sensationalist media reports about problem doctors could easily erode one's confidence in doctors and the medical profession. But I remain optimistic about the patient–doctor relationship. There are many encouraging signs. More and more patients are seeking to be actively engaged in their own health care, and doctors are increasingly working in partnership with them. Patients report high levels of satisfaction with their own doctor, and the public scores doctors very highly in polls of trusted professionals. It seems that most of us encounter good doctors when we need medical care.

Why, then, write a book about good doctors and patient expectations, if the overall picture is fairly rosy? I want to reflect on my own experience as an arbiter of patient complaints, and to suggest some areas for improvement. I have seen first-hand how patients and doctors relate to each other in New Zealand. I have helped draft and interpret the laws governing their relationship, and have contributed to ethical guidelines and policy developments impacting on it. I have had the privilege of researching health policy and medical regulation in the United States, Canada, the United Kingdom and Australia.[1] I have seen wonderful examples of innovation in health policy and patient care in New Zealand – but also areas where patient expectations and medical practice lag behind comparable countries. I want to share the lessons I have learnt.

I also bring my personal background to my writing. I do not come from a professional family, and have rarely been a patient. I am trained in law, not medicine. But I have long been interested in how people get cared for when they become patients, and intrigued by doctors and what makes them tick. I find the patient–doctor relationship fascinating.

Background

My first real contact with the world of medicine came in the 1980s, when my youngest brother studied medicine and commenced work as a house surgeon in a provincial hospital in New Zealand. I was surprised when he told me occasional stories of consultants known within the hospital community to be substandard. My young doctor friends told me similar stories. I found this surprising, but it did not occupy me greatly at the time. I was busy with my own studies and career. To the extent I gave the matter any thought at all, I admired the young students who attained the high grades needed to study medicine, and was fascinated by the skills they acquired and the diverse and intimate roles they assumed. Medicine, I thought, was a privileged profession.

Fast-forward to the year 2000. I had just been appointed as New Zealand's Health and Disability Commissioner (HDC), a national health ombudsman responsible for handling complaints about health care and disability services. I now had a 'public watchdog' role, charged with promoting and protecting patients' rights in New Zealand. Complaints about doctors whose care or communication was alleged to be substandard featured prominently in HDC's work.

Over the intervening two decades, I had spent a brief period in legal practice, before working as a legal academic in Canada, the United States and New Zealand. I had developed an interest in medical ethics and started a new course in medico-legal issues at Auckland University. In the 1990s, this took me into the world of health management in New Zealand (including a stint at the Northern Regional Health Authority, where I contributed to the development of priority access criteria for the end stage renal failure programme), and health policy and regulation (as manager of mental health policy and regulation, and later Deputy Director-General, Safety and Regulation, at the Ministry of Health).

I worked as an advisor on the drafting of the first modern health practitioner statute in New Zealand (the Medical Practitioners Act 1995). I witnessed the political power of organised medicine during that parliamentary process, and later in the successful lobbying to have the criminal law amended (by the Crimes Amendment Act 1997), in response to the prosecution of several doctors for manslaughter where patients had died following medical negligence. I helped draft New Zealand's Code of Health and Disability Services Consumers' Rights 1996 – pioneering legislation giving patients (and other consumers of health and disability services) legally enforceable rights,[2] enacted in response to a public inquiry report revealing individual and systemic failures in the treatment of women with cervical carcinoma *in situ* at National Women's Hospital in Auckland in the 1960s and 1970s.

Thus, by the year 2000, I was well versed in health practitioner regulation, familiar with the influence of the medical profession, and aware of the ability of doctors to do great good, but also to cause significant harm. I began my work as Commissioner with a healthy respect for the skills and dedication of the vast majority of doctors. I left office in 2010, confirmed in my view that we are generally very well served by the professionalism of modern doctors.

A perplexing problem
But in my work as Commissioner, in handling thousands of complaints about health practitioners, and the systems in which they worked, one issue emerged periodically and gnawed away at me: the poorly performing practitioner. It became clear to me that, despite supposed safeguards, some incompetent practitioners were able to continue in practice and harm patients. More worryingly, I observed the apparent unwillingness or inability of regulators to take any decisive action to improve the situation.

The incompetent doctor was the practitioner who gave me most reason for concern. Time and again, I saw cases where it must (or should) have been apparent to colleagues, may well have been suspected by patients, and would probably have been detected by thorough checks by a medical regulator, that a doctor was performing inadequately. Equally concerning, I saw cases where even reactive checking (following complaints and concerns) led to very limited assessment of a doctor's performance.

I found this situation was unsatisfactory. I was not comforted by the knowledge that systems, rather than individuals, are the underlying cause of most healthcare-induced harm, nor by bland assurances from medical authorities and politicians that the current system for protecting the public was adequate. I realised that concerns notified to safety agencies and medical regulators were likely to be the tip of the iceberg.

Estimates of the prevalence of substandard medical practice are very difficult to obtain, partly because regular periodic assessment of ongoing competence does not occur. Most experts agree that 1 to 2 per cent of current doctors are probably not practising at an acceptable level; some privately concede that the figure may be as high as 5 per cent.[3] Similar figures have been suggested to me in discussions with medical regulators in the United Kingdom, the United States, Canada, Australia and New Zealand. Accepting that most doctors, perhaps around 95 per cent, are self-motivated to keep up to date, and do provide an appropriate standard of care, that still leaves 600 doctors (in New Zealand's population of approximately 12,000 doctors) who may be providing inadequate care. We do not know where the bar is, given the lack of agreed standards in many areas of medicine, nor how many practitioners fall below it.

This problem crosses jurisdictional boundaries. In my contact with overseas health ombudsmen and medical regulators, I learnt that other health and legal systems fail to detect incompetent doctors before patients are harmed, and that rigorous checks are seldom undertaken before (and sometimes even after) problems arise. Too often, the end result of such cases is that a patient receives substandard care and may be harmed, the doctor suffers the shame and ignominy of external investigations and, in extreme cases, there is a loss of trust in the medical profession and in the regulators charged with protecting the public.

This was brought home to me most clearly when, in 2004, I was called as an expert to a seminar in Manchester, England on regulation and complaints, held as part of the Shipman Inquiry: the inquiry into the career of GP Harold Shipman, who murdered over 200 of his patients. Later, I read Dame Janet Smith's excoriating criticism, in her final report, of the planned system for revalidating doctors in the United Kingdom. How could something seemingly so simple – checking that licensed doctors remain competent and fit to practise – be so difficult?

The more I talked to people responsible for overseeing doctors' ongoing competence, and to doctors themselves, and the more I read about the topic, the clearer it became that ensuring a doctor's ongoing competence is not easy. Nor is the challenge a new one. In the novel *The Citadel*,[4] a popular classic published in 1937, an aspiring young Scottish doctor commences practice in the remote mining valleys of Wales. He decries the outdated methods of his fellow doctors: 'There ought to be a law to make doctors keep up to date. It's all the fault of our rotten system. There ought to be compulsory post-graduate classes – to be taken every five years . . .'

There have undoubtedly been improvements in the intervening 75 years. Today, laws that seek to mandate medical competence are generally in place, and CME (continuing medical education) and CPD (continuing professional development) is well entrenched. Yet whether doctors stay up to date is still predominantly a matter of individual conscience, and whether their efforts translate into good practice is seldom subject to rigorous checks. This fact is well known amongst doctors, but comes as a surprise to most members of the public.

Good doctors and patient expectations

This book is my attempt to explain why the simple aim of ensuring that every licensed doctor is a good doctor has proven so difficult to achieve – and to suggest the steps that need to be taken to meet the modest expectations of patients. It is divided into four parts: the ideal, the reality, the roadblocks, and a prescription for change.

I point to changes occurring internationally (particularly in the areas of transparent, readily accessible information for patients, and checking of doctors' competence) and their implications for medical practice, especially in New Zealand and Australia. I suggest some concrete steps that should be taken to build trust between the public and the medical profession. I argue for a model of good medical practice that will realise the legitimate expectations of patients, encourage true professionalism in doctors, and form the basis of a new contract between patients and doctors.

I advocate for changes in the areas of information, competence and trust. Patients deserve better information about doctors (and the health service) and an assurance of medical competence. I want patients to know what to expect when they seek medical care, and to be encouraged to speak up when their information needs and expectations of competent care are not met. I want doctors to be persuaded by the case for more information and enhanced competence checks, but also to be helped to make any necessary changes to their practice and the way they currently maintain competence. If people see evidence of a modern medical profession whose members are committed to demonstrating ongoing competence, there will be a good basis for continued public trust in the profession.

Other actors have an important role to play in achieving change. I encourage consumer advocacy groups to lobby for the changes proposed in this book. I hope politicians and policy-makers will see the opportunity for an improved health service, and take action to support it. I urge medical educators to place greater emphasis on patient expectations and the responsibilities of modern doctors. I want funders of health care and doctors' employers to support the information agenda and the implementation of more effective and consistent credentialling processes. For colleges and medical specialist societies, the challenge is to develop enhanced continuing professional development tools, and to support Fellows in new ways of maintaining competence, with clear expectations that they do so.[5]

My original intention was to write a book confined to the specific issue of recertification of doctors. It forms a key part of my prescription for change. But I also want medical regulators to shift from being inwardly focused on the medical profession. Medical boards need to become much more outward looking, providing clear information to the public about the steps being taken to promote patient safety and ensure doctors remain competent. Greater transparency from regulators, and more rigorous recertification and competence review processes, will help maintain public confidence in the medical profession and its watchdogs.

There will always be sad tales of patients harmed when things go wrong in health care. They usually come to public notice because unhappy patients and families (often frustrated by the official response to their concerns) want to tell their story, and it feeds a public interest. But media reporting can easily foster public distrust, with sensationalist stories of medical misdiagnoses, surgical 'botch-ups' and dodgy doctors. One final hope in writing this book is to encourage responsible health journalists to dig deeper – to become better informed about patient expectations and developments in health policy internationally, and the positive changes being made by many doctors and medical groups, and to bring those stories to public notice.

Why doctors and why patients?

Another writer might easily choose to write about health providers of all types, and health consumers. Many of the issues raised in this book are of broader application than simply to doctors and patients. Why have I chosen to focus on doctors, through the lens of patients?

In the developed world, we are all likely to be cared for by a doctor at some point during our lives. The majority of us have a regular doctor, but the relationship is unlike most of our other professional dealings. We often see our doctor when we are feeling unwell, not at our best, and we can easily feel disempowered and assume the attitude of a supplicant, even though we (or the State on our behalf) are usually paying for the service. Unless we have become an expert in the health problem about which we are seeking the doctor's advice, we probably have less knowledge about the issue, and are dependent on the skills and knowledge of the practitioner.

Such dependency and power imbalance is true in many situations where we seek professional advice. Yet we are not expected to bare our bodies for other professional advisors to examine. We share intimate details of our personal lives with our doctor – something we may also do when consulting a lawyer, accountant or pastor, but without the overlay of fears about ill health and mortality that sometimes hover in the doctor's surgery. We may not believe that doctors have special healing powers, but even the modern general practitioner may be seen as a 'suburban shaman' (in the words of doctor anthropologist Cecil Helman).[6]

Although no longer put on a pedestal by the general populace, doctors still occupy positions of relative privilege and prestige in the community. In an age of obsession with health and wellbeing, their special knowledge is highly valued and their opinions are widely cited. Doctors are glamorised in movies and on TV, and demonised in the media when they harm or exploit their patients. Heroes or villains, they matter to us.

Many of the messages in this book are relevant for other health professions. Our relationship with some other health practitioners – notably midwives and nurses – may share the patient–doctor characteristics of vulnerability and intimacy, and depend on effective communication for the best results. Modern health systems increasingly rely on service delivery by skilled non-medical practitioners, who are accorded status as independent practitioners with special privileges. As with doctors, we want to know that nurses, midwives, dentists, pharmacists, optometrists and other health practitioners also remain competent; we expect them to be trustworthy and to provide us with the information we need about their services.

But as a society, we accord greater status to doctors, and we place higher expectations on medical practitioners. In a health crisis, our first port of call will usually be a doctor. Doctors regularly take ultimate responsibility for medical decisions and diagnoses in situations of complexity and uncertainty.[7] As members of the public, we tend to give doctors primacy in the ranks of health practitioners. Certainly, when things go wrong in health care, doctors are the group most often complained about by patients.[8] Doctors enjoy special attention from health politicians and funders. And whenever health reforms are mooted, the medical profession shows a determination to stay at the top of the totem pole of healthcare delivery.

A key focus of the book is the poorly performing practitioner who fails to meet patient expectations. One might ask in response, why single out the individual health practitioner? If most problems in healthcare delivery occur because of a breakdown in systems, and we want to improve safety and quality, shouldn't we concentrate our efforts in that direction?

Focusing on the role of individuals working in the healthcare system can be seen as an outmoded way of thinking that all too easily leads to finger-pointing, blame and shame.

The emphasis on fixing faulty systems is laudable – and probably where we will get most bang for our buck in investing in healthcare quality improvement. Yet it is not the whole story. The individual practitioners working in the system are critical to patients receiving good care and information. A competent doctor may be unable to overcome the defects in a healthcare delivery system, but an incompetent doctor can frustrate the best care system in the world, causing preventable harm or wasting the time and energy of other health practitioners, who learn to 'work around' the problem. Patients are dependent on the clinical and communication skills of their individual doctor.

I have also deliberately chosen to write of patients. I know that some people dislike being called a patient, because of connotations of suffering[9] and passivity. They prefer a word that emphasises that doctors are providing a service that they are using, and often paying for. I prefer the old-fashioned word, patient, because it's how most people describe themselves when they consult a doctor in the community, or are seen by a doctor in hospital.[10] I may be a client of my physiotherapist, and a user or consumer of disability services, but when I see a doctor, I'm happy to be called a patient. I know that it's a word that works for doctors too, many of whom bristle slightly when people start talking about consumers,[11] users or clients, and don't warm to being called providers.

Good intentions are not enough

What is my approach in writing this book about good doctors and patient expectations, and in analysing the patient–doctor relationship more generally? I accept that the vast majority of doctors are well intentioned. They go to work to care for their patients – to diagnose illness, offer treatment where possible, and relieve suffering. They aspire to be 'good doctors', in accordance with the codes of 'good medical practice' adopted by the medical profession in the United Kingdom, Canada, Australia and New Zealand.

But good intentions are not enough. As a member of the public, and a potential patient, I want to know that I can rely on the public medical register and the simple fact of a current licence to practise medicine as assurance that any licensed doctor is competent. I find it unacceptable that, within the medical community, it is often common knowledge that a certain doctor should be avoided for the care of one's own family, but that the general public is not privy to such information. I accept that within any profession there will always be outliers: the gifted and the ordinary. I want to know that even the ordinary practitioner meets minimum standards.

I appreciate that doctors already feel overregulated, and that a balance needs to be found between relying exclusively on professionalism and self-regulation on the one hand, and external regulation on the other. I have always seen the role of the law in this area as being to promote, not hinder, the delivery of good-quality health care. But the law also exists to protect individuals, and in my view we have erred too far on the side of light-handed regulation. We have trusted but not verified.

I hope the messages in this book will strike a chord with patients and doctors. I want my ideas to prompt debate and lead to change.

1

THE GOOD DOCTOR
THE IDEAL

In this part of the book, I seek to describe the ideal situation, in which patient expectations of receiving care from a good doctor are routinely fulfilled. I explain what I mean by a good doctor, based on the views of patients and doctors themselves. I introduce the concept of the 'good enough' doctor, who may not be excellent but who fulfils our expectations, in contrast to the 'problem doctor', who does not reach this threshold. Finally, I explain how, in an ideal world, patients would be able to rest easy in the assurance that every licensed doctor is a good doctor.

What is a good doctor?

'Patients need good doctors', proclaims the General Medical Council (the statutory body that has regulated doctors in the United Kingdom since 1858) in the opening statement of its guidance for doctors, *Good Medical Practice*.[1] 'Everyone is entitled to a good doctor', states Donald Irvine, paraphrasing William Osler, the acclaimed scholar and teacher who was said to epitomise a good doctor at the start of the twentieth century.[2] 'Most doctors are good doctors in the eyes of most patients', writes health advocate Angela Coulter.[3] The phrase is bandied about in the health policy and sociology literature about doctors, and in the media when individual doctors are praised for their community service, or defended by patients in the face of official sanctions for misdeeds.[4]

In his powerful novel *The Good Doctor*, author Damon Galgut contrasts the characters of two doctors, one deeply cynical yet realistic, the other naively optimistic and seeking to do good, in remote, rural post-apartheid South Africa.[5] The reader is left to ponder whether either of these flawed men is a good doctor. The word 'good' when applied to doctors is ambiguous, speaking both to the motivation and character of the workers, but also to the quality of their work. This ambiguity is reflected in attempts to define the attributes of a good doctor, and to describe the characteristics of good medical practice. Invariably, the desired qualities relate to both motivation and performance. The duality is also seen in an influential seventeenth-century definition of a physician as *vir bonus medicinae peritus*, a good man expert in medicine.[6]

Governments, insurers and employers, as funders of medical care, are interested in what makes a good doctor. So, too, are the medical schools and colleges that train doctors, the medical professional organisations that seek to promote the interests of doctors, and the regulators charged with overseeing medical practice. The ultimate arbiter, of course, should be the patients on the receiving end of medical care.

Patients' views

Individual patients form their own views about what to look for in a doctor, influenced by personal experience and the experience of friends and family. With the burgeoning literature about doctors and health, some patients may even be primed in how to get the best out of their doctor, and alert to pitfalls in medical practice.[7]

Patient associations represent patients' views in advocating for the standards of care and practice they expect of doctors. Health researchers, health policy and advocacy organisations, medical associations, medical regulators, and funders periodically undertake surveys and debate what patients look for in doctors. In the discussion that follows I have drawn on published surveys and literature from such groups. My thinking is also influenced by my observations from reading hundreds of letters from patients about their doctor, in which they praise great care and lament failings.

Technical competence

Patients generally rate technical competence as the most important attribute in a doctor. By 'technical' competence I mean the knowledge, training and experience to provide an appropriate level of medical care and the practical skills to do so. Some researchers draw a distinction between 'competence' (knowing what to do) and 'performance' (doing it),[8] but I doubt that the general public makes this distinction. People expect both in their doctor. Competence in communication is obviously an important aspect of broader clinical competence, but patients generally differentiate between 'bedside manner' and knowledge or 'technical' competence.

Patients understand that doctors are cogs in a complex health system, and that sometimes things go wrong in health care. Public reports and media coverage of 'serious and sentinel events' causing harm to hospital patients have become relatively routine.[9] The public is also used to being told, in the wake of human tragedy in many settings, that the outcome was caused by a 'systems' problem. However, in my experience, people are sceptical about the claim that the vast majority of unintended harm to patients is caused by faulty systems, not incompetent individuals – at least when asked to apply that general proposition to a specific case. The public and the media look for an individual practitioner to be held accountable.

Even if we accept the key role of safe systems in delivering safe care, the technical competence of individual health practitioners, especially doctors (who are often in the driving seat), remains a crucial factor. As Nancy Berlinger writes: 'Mistakes are made by individuals, even if these individuals are working within systems.'[10] Patients expect their individual doctor to be skilled and competent, and are wary of experts who glibly invoke the 'systems' mantra in the aftermath of disaster.

Public surveys and submissions from patient advocacy groups confirm this expectation. In a 2009 survey of 289 customers of 10 pharmacies in Dunedin, competence was ranked as the number one professional attribute for a doctor.[11] In a 2006 submission, the Federation of Women's Health Councils Aotearoa New Zealand noted that patients expect a '[h]igh level of medical competence – good up-to-date medical knowledge and diagnostic skills, sound technique for medical procedures and awareness of limitations'.[12] In a 2010 survey of 502 members of the New Zealand public, 97 per cent agreed with the statement that it is essential that doctors stay up to date with developments in medicine.[13]

THE IDEAL

(Hardly surprising – indeed it's intriguing that 100 per cent didn't agree with such a leading statement, and that 1 per cent 'strongly disagreed' with the proposition!)

Of course, most patients have no knowledge of a doctor's training (at best they may notice a faded degree certificate on the surgery wall), experience, or current skills. Unless a doctor is obviously inept at history taking, examination and diagnosis, it is difficult for patients to judge their competence – though an expert patient may sense that something is amiss. In *A Fortunate Man*, a moving account of an English country doctor in the 1960s, John Berger writes: 'You have to be a startlingly bad doctor and make many mistakes before the results tell against you. In the eyes of the layman the results always tend to favour the doctor.'[14]

As a general rule, in the words of Donald Irvine, 'although patients can judge a doctor's personal qualities, they have to take clinical competence on trust because they cannot assess it satisfactorily'.[15] Patients assume that their doctor knows what to do, and can do the job competently. They appreciate that medicine is complex and that sometimes specialist advice is needed. They expect doctors to recognise the limits of their own professional competence and refer to another practitioner if they are out of their depth.

Putting patients first

Technical competence is only part of the equation. Patients also value other professional and personal qualities in a medical practitioner. If asked, members of the public list a wide range of desired non-technical attributes. One key quality is whether the doctor makes the care of the patient his or her first concern. In a survey of 98 members of the public undertaken by the Picker Institute in England in 2006, this was rated as the most important duty of a doctor by 78 per cent of respondents.[16]

How are patients to judge whether a doctor places their best interests first? It is something that patients take for granted and are not well placed to assess. There may be glaring examples of a doctor being distracted and not focusing on the current patient – for example, interrupting the consultation to take a non-urgent cellphone call about a business matter.[17] In the absence of obvious omissions to give primacy to their interests, patients will assume that they are the main focus of the doctor's attention. They *trust* this to be the case.

Patients understand that there are competing demands on doctors' time. They are generally tolerant of having to wait, but if the doctor says a referral letter will be sent, or test results will be reviewed and the patient contacted if there is anything untoward, naturally the patient assumes that this will happen. So, if a doctor is indifferent or lax in these areas of professional responsibility, the patient will feel let down; that their care has not, after all, been the doctor's first concern.

Many instances of failing to give primacy to patients' interests will be covert. If a doctor provides unconventional treatment in pursuance of his own research theory, without his patients' knowledge or consent – as Dr Herbert Green did at National Women's Hospital in the events uncovered in the Cartwright Inquiry[18] – they will feel betrayed when they later learn the true situation, however good his intentions. Similarly, if a surgeon takes an unnecessary biopsy for research purposes, without the patient's informed consent,[19] performs unnecessary stent operations,[20] or orders unwarranted tests for extraneous purposes (such as meeting a funder's target), the patient is likely to feel aggrieved. Such behaviour is not consistent with good medical practice, and even if the doctor claims to be well motivated, any avowal to be a good doctor is undermined by their failure to make the care of the patient their first concern.

Integrity and trustworthiness

Patients expect integrity and trustworthiness in their doctor. In the Dunedin survey cited above, being trustworthy and honest with patients scored just below competence as the most highly valued professional attributes. Like competence and putting patients first, professional integrity is something that patients assume but cannot easily judge for themselves. When a doctor is revealed to have betrayed a patient's trust, both the conduct and the character of the doctor are likely to be criticised.

One obvious type of dishonesty is financial exploitation: the doctor who overcharges, receives an undisclosed kickback from a specialist or private facility to whom they made a referral, or sees the patient for a fee in private without disclosing the option of a free consultation in the public system.[21] A more common example of untrustworthy behaviour is disclosing only the doctor's preferred treatment intervention, or failing to disclose that an injury or complication resulted from a medical mistake. Breach of confidentiality, such as the doctor who divulges the patient's private confidences outside the consultation room as gossip, rather than for purposes of treatment, is also a breach of trust.

More extreme examples of dishonesty and violation of trust are the physician who undertakes unnecessary procedures to provide cover for prescribing restricted medicines to which the doctor is addicted; the sexual predator who undertakes unnecessary physical examinations for personal gratification or who sexually assaults the patient; and the murderous doctor who kills an unsuspecting patient under the guise of medical treatment.

All of the above examples, to varying degrees, involve a breach of trust in which the doctor's personal interests are advanced at the patient's expense. Doctors who behave in this way, and are caught out, almost invariably face disciplinary process and professional censure, and may incur criminal penalties. Their behaviour is unlawful and unethical, and calls into question their integrity and moral character.

There is some survey evidence that the public is tolerant of misdemeanours in the private lives of doctors, so long as this doesn't spill over into their professional work. This is reflected in modern medical regulation, with statutes removing requirements that relate to the 'good character' of the doctor. However, criminal behaviour in a doctor's personal life (such as domestic abuse or accessing child pornography) is likely to result in professional discipline, since such conduct reflects on whether the doctor is a 'fit and proper person' to practise medicine.

Communication skills
One aspect of clinical competence that matters highly to patients, and that they are well placed to judge, is whether the doctor is a good communicator. Right 5(1) of the New Zealand Code of Health and Disability Services Consumers' Rights affirms the right 'to effective communication in a form, language, and manner that enables the consumer to understand the information provided'.[22] From my experience, it will often be an aspect of the doctor's communication or manner, rather than a simple mistake, that will trigger a patient's complaint. If a doctor 'talks down' to a patient, or fails to explain clinical terms or to attempt to answer a patient's questions, miscommunication is all but guaranteed, and the stage set for a complaint if things go wrong. Research indicates a correlation between good doctor–patient communication and improved patient health outcomes.[23]

There are many elements of effective communication between patients and doctors. Patients care about whether their doctor listens, engages with them, provides helpful information and explanations, and spends adequate time with them during the consultation. A European study in 2002 listed top patient priorities in primary care as having enough time in the consultation, and having a general practitioner who listens and provides helpful information about their illness and treatment options, and encourages them to discuss all their problems. Levinson and Pizzo note that patients in Canada and the United States often find their physician 'too busy to listen and too distant to care'.[24]

In our early meetings with any new professional advisor – often during the opening moments of a consultation – we generally make a rapid assessment of whether they are a good communicator. Given the intimate nature of the professional relationship between patients and doctors, the ability to communicate well is especially important. A skilful doctor is able to give the patient enough time to warm up and feel comfortable explaining the reason for the consultation, and then to focus the discussion on key issues and to elicit the information necessary to form a diagnosis or determine next steps. A doctor who is a good communicator will try to ensure that the patient does not leave the surgery with unanswered questions; will explain how to contact the doctor again with any follow-up questions that do not require another face-to-face consultation; will tell the patient about any concerning side effects or changes to watch out for, and what to do; and will provide practical instructions on any next steps (such as getting test results).

Many of the matters discussed under the rubric of communication are pivotal to whether a patient feels fully involved in their own care, and able to play a full part in a 'therapeutic partnership' with the doctor. Patient involvement and engagement has been a major theme in the patient–doctor literature in the past decade.[25] The twenty-first century has been called 'the century of the patient', and the hallmark of the evolving patient–doctor relationship is said to be shared decision-making. As Martin Marshall notes, this involves a 're-conceptualisation of the role and responsibilities of patients and health professionals in improving health', with the interaction 'increasingly being framed as a meeting between two experts', something that runs counter to the traditional culture of medicine.[26] Not all patients will want this level of involvement, but most will appreciate being asked how much input they want to have into their own medical care, so that the ground rules for the relationship are clear.

The General Medical Council's guidance on consent endorses shared decision-making as the norm for most medical decisions:

> Whatever the context in which medical decisions are made, you must work in partnership with your patients to ensure good care. In so doing, you must:

a. listen to patients and respect their views about their health
b. discuss with patients what their diagnosis, prognosis, treatment and care involve
c. share with patients the information they want or need in order to make decisions
d. maximise patients' opportunities, and their ability, to make decisions for themselves
e. respect patients' decisions.[27]

Finally, an important but less visible element of a doctor's communication skills is how effectively he or she maintains patient records, makes referrals to other practitioners, and communicates with professional colleagues. Most patients never see their own records or, if they do, lack the clinical knowledge and the familiarity necessary to interpret them and make comparisons with other clinical records. Any medico-legal inquirer soon learns that accurate and meaningful records are an essential part of the patient's story, helping to guide future care. Records are a vital aspect of good care, as well as enabling audit and research. Poor records are often a pointer to other problems in a doctor's practice.

When a doctor's referral letters or order forms for tests and procedures are unclear or omit key clinical information, the poor communication is a potential barrier to quality care. So, too, if a doctor is rude or uncommunicative with colleagues, or unwilling to pick up the phone and find out why a referral is delayed, or what's happening with a patient's care, the stage will be set for problems. Patients need their doctors to be effective advocates, and that entails being a good communicator with all the other practitioners involved in their care.

New Zealand's Code of Health and Disability Services Consumers' Rights contains a curiously worded provision, right 4(5), which states that '[e]very consumer has the right to co-operation among providers to ensure quality and continuity of services'. The wording is inapt, since although co-operation among providers (particularly between different professional groups, such as doctors and midwives) is important, co-ordination of the care provided by multiple providers is also essential. In practice, right 4(5) has proved invaluable in highlighting problems in care co-ordination.[28] For care to be co-ordinated, the left hand needs to know what the right hand is doing. A doctor who fails to communicate effectively with colleagues provides fertile ground for discontinuity of care, and falls short on an important indicator of being a good doctor.

Respect and caring
Patients also highly value 'humaneness' in their doctor – qualities such as respect and caring. It is no accident that the right to be treated with respect is the first of the 10 rights affirmed in New Zealand's Code. During consultations in 1995 on the draft Code, community groups highlighted the importance of respectful treatment of patients. The final Code provision covers basic respect, respect for privacy, and respect for the needs, values and beliefs of different cultural, religious, social and ethnic groups.[29] Provision of services in a manner that respects individual dignity and independence is also a legal right under the New Zealand Code.[30] The new Constitution of the National Health Service in England similarly states that patients are legally entitled to be treated with dignity and respect.[31]

If respect is the bottom line, caring – kindness, courtesy and compassion – is what many patients yearn for. They are frequently disappointed. Whether for reasons of work pressure, bureaucratic demands, changing patterns of healthcare delivery, or endemic culture, the absence of compassion in the health system is a concern commonly expressed by patients and their families – and by stressed health practitioners working in the system.[32] It is a concern being voiced in health systems all around the world.

Patients in New Zealand value care and attentiveness from their doctor. The Nationwide Health & Disability Consumer Advocacy Service from 2006 onwards asked people to send in accounts of great care. The resulting publication, *The Art of Great Care: Stories from people who have experienced great care*,[33] is revealing. Often, it is the small signs of caring that really make a difference. A partially sighted woman describes her general practitioner as a 'doctor who really cares'.[34] Her doctor is attentive to her needs: 'waits for me in the reception area, to make sure I have heard her call, and can find my way to her room'. Her GP is respectful: 'doesn't focus on my disability unless it is relevant to the health issue I am facing right then'. Most of all, her doctor shows that she cares: 'although very busy, she has taken the trouble to put herself in my shoes, and to treat me as a whole human being, with courtesy and imagination'.

Caring is a quality that many patients especially appreciate in times of illness and worry. Essayist Anatole Broyard, facing metastatic prostatic cancer, wrote: 'I'd like my doctor to scan me, to grope for my spirit as well as my prostate. Without some recognition, I am nothing but my illness.'[35] Broyard wished that his doctor would 'give me his whole mind just once, be bonded with me for a brief space, survey my soul as well as my flesh'.[36]

The qualities of kindness and caring are relevant not only to the good deeds that a doctor performs, but also to the attitude that accompanies the acts. A doctor who is competent, patient-centred, trustworthy and an effective communicator is, from an objective viewpoint, a good doctor. Yet if that same doctor displays these qualities while maintaining clinical detachment and brisk efficiency, some patients may feel that something is missing: the fellow feeling and caring approach that many patients describe when recalling a good doctor. Physician and writer Rafael Campo describes a remarkable AIDS patient, Gary, who in 'the availability of his suffering' helps Campo 'remove the mask' he wears in hospital and brings him closer to the suffering of his patients.[37]

Patients may understand the reasons for a doctor's detachment, and may even find it more comfortable to keep the relationship on an entirely professional footing. Yet many patients hold on to the ideal of a healing relationship, and draw comfort and reassurance from small signs that the doctor has the moral character and imagination to stand in their shoes for a moment. John Sassall, the country doctor observed in *A Fortunate Man*, is acknowledged by his patients 'as a good doctor because he meets the deep but unformulated expectation of the sick for a sense of fraternity'.[38]

Doctors' views

It's hardly surprising that the views of patients are echoed in the opinions of doctors themselves. As health professionals, doctors observe the qualities to be found in a well-rounded doctor – and appreciate that good doctors come in different guises. In addition to their professional perspective, many doctors have insights from being a patient, especially as they age.[39]

Doctors know that both technical competence and humanistic qualities are essential attributes of the complete doctor. Bioethicist and medical historian Albert Jonsen describes competence as 'the essential, the comprehensive virtue' of modern medicine, noting that writings from the sixteenth and seventeenth centuries on the duties of physicians repeat as the first imperative: 'Let the physician be competent.'[40] A book published in 1684 claimed that the first mortal sin of physicians is 'practising medicine without being thoroughly competent in the art'.[41]

By the early twentieth century, in response to the growing emphasis on clinical competence and the scientific basis of medicine, some voices within the medical profession reminded colleagues of the need for humanity as well as technical skill. Harvard physician Francis Peabody famously declared: '[T]he secret of the care of the patient is in caring for the patient.'[42] Compassion has long been identified, in eastern and western medicine, as a virtue in a doctor. The seventh-century Chinese physician Sun Simiao described the Ideal Physician as one who develops 'a heart of great mercy and compassion'.[43] The twelfth-century Jewish philosopher-physician Maimonides also identified the need for fellow feeling in the medical practitioner. He prayed: 'May I never forget that the patient is a fellow creature in pain. May I never consider him merely a vessel of disease.'[44]

Both qualities – competence and compassion – are proclaimed as essential virtues by contemporary doctors. In a *British Medical Journal* debate in 2002 about what makes a good doctor, readers from 24 countries emphasised personal qualities ahead of proficiency in knowledge and technical skills. This duality is reflected in the Code of Conduct issued in 2010 by the Medical Board of Australia. It states: 'Patients trust their doctors because they believe that, in addition to being competent, their doctor will not take advantage of them and will display qualities such as integrity, truthfulness, dependability and compassion.'[45]

The Hippocratic Oath, which dates from the fourth century BC, makes no mention of competence or compassion, but Jonsen observes that '[i]f anything deserves the title "Hippocratic ethic" it is the imperative of competent practice of the art'.[46] He traces the adoption of medicine as a university subject and a guild activity in the Middle Ages as the time when 'competence became a notable and explicit virtue'.[47] Modern codes of ethics identify both competence and compassion as the primary virtues. The American Medical Association Code of Medical Ethics states, as its first principle: 'A physician shall be dedicated to providing competent medical care, with compassion and respect for human dignity and rights.'[48]

A discussion of doctors' views of what it means to be a good doctor would not be complete without a brief discussion of what it means to be a medical *professional*. The idea of belonging to a profession, and the concept of professionalism, inform how doctors think.

The profession and professionalism

Doctors are proud to be members of a learned profession. Many doctors claim to have a vocation to practise medicine. They do not see themselves as mere service providers such as plumbers and drainlayers, who also offer their specialised knowledge and skills on a fee-for-service basis to members of the public, and must be licensed to do so. Although other providers, such as gasfitters and air traffic controllers, also work in areas where public safety is paramount, unlike doctors they are not usually described as members of a profession.

Sociologist Eliot Freidson, in his classic work *Profession of Medicine*,[49] defined a profession as a work group that is given the right to control its own work. Freidson identified the hallmarks of a profession as (1) expertise, the possession of special skills and knowledge; (2) altruism or commitment to public service; and (3) self-scrutiny or the freedom to self-regulate.

How does this translate into practice in medicine? The cumulative effect of a specialised, arcane body of knowledge, the antiquity of the practice of the medicine, the peculiar vulnerability of patients, and the right to monopoly practice and to self-regulate, differentiate medicine (and, by analogy, other professions such as law, accountancy and engineering) from other common callings. The State (via the legislature) grants doctors the exclusive right to work as medical practitioners, and (to varying degrees) the right to self-regulate. Within their lawful scope of practice, doctors are free to exercise a large degree of clinical autonomy in making decisions about patient care.

However, the freedom of the profession to regulate itself is coming under pressure. In the wake of public scandals where the profession is seen not to have kept its house in order, the emphasis has shifted to accountability. Commentators note that the privilege of self-regulation 'entails an absolute obligation to guarantee the competence of members. The setting and maintenance of standards is of overriding importance, and issues such as recertification and revalidation are, without question, now regarded as professional obligations.'[50] Scandals involving 'bad apples' in the profession represent 'a failure in the profession's guarantee that each of its members would be trustworthy as to competence and character' and provoke and legitimise the collapse of self-regulation.[51]

If expertise, altruism and self-regulation are features of a profession, what does it mean to be a professional? I have often been struck by how readily, in the presence of medical practitioners, a discussion about the role of the doctor segues into a conversation about the importance of professionalism. (An earnest discussion of medical leadership often follows in a group of male doctors over the age of forty!) Professionalism is an article of faith for most doctors. It is seen as the basis of the medical profession's implicit contract with society. At its best, professionalism is a commitment by members of a profession to maintain high standards and serve the public, in return for the privileges accorded to its practitioners.

But professionalism is under threat. 'Consumerism is outpacing the social contract of professionalism', claims quality expert Don Berwick.[52] Certainly, professionalism is not a term that resonates with members of the public. It has unfashionable connotations of exclusivity and clubbiness. Ian Kennedy's passing reference to the 'club culture' at Bristol Royal Infirmary was one of the most cited parts of the Bristol Inquiry report, even though the report contained many positive references to the medical profession.[53] Any perception of an insular, self-serving profession, closed to outsiders, is corrosive of public trust. I recall Harvard professor of medicine David Blumenthal warning that professionalism can be 'a refuge of scoundrels'.[54] If members of a profession take refuge behind a cloak of professionalism to defend questionable practices, trust is swiftly eroded.

Professional leaders are sensitive to such criticisms. In 2001, physician groups on both sides of the Atlantic launched a new charter entitled 'Medical Professionalism in the New Millennium', in an attempt to restate the profession's commitment to public service. In North America, the charter originated in part from a sense that the medical profession was under siege, especially from financial incentives on doctors. While those factors were less pressing in the publicly funded Antipodean health systems, the lofty principles of the new charter of medical professionalism were enthusiastically endorsed by medical associations and leading doctors.[55]

The first of three 'fundamental principles' expressed in the physicians' charter is primacy of patient welfare (the other two are patient autonomy and social justice). Ten professional responsibilities are listed in the charter. The first is a strong statement of the importance of maintaining professional competence: 'Physicians must be committed to lifelong learning and be responsible for maintaining the medical knowledge and clinical and team skills necessary for the provision of quality care. More broadly, the profession as a whole must strive to see that all of its members are competent and must ensure that appropriate mechanisms are available for physicians to accomplish this goal.' The second responsibility is a commitment to honesty with patients.

Of course, just because doctors espouse high-minded principles doesn't mean that they are followed in practice. In response to a survey in 2003, 1662 medical specialists in the United States reported high levels of support for the aspirations in the physicians' charter. Yet there were notable gaps between doctors' beliefs and what they reported doing. For example, 96 per cent of respondents believed physicians should report all instances of significantly impaired or incompetent colleagues to their hospital, clinic or other relevant authorities; yet almost one half of physicians who were aware of an impaired or incompetent colleague did not bring that doctor to the attention of authorities.[56]

Putting to one side this discordance between rhetoric and reality, it is clear that declarations from the medical profession are consistent with patients' views of what makes a good doctor. The desired qualities are well summarised by Donald Irvine, who writes:

> When patients and their relatives say they have a 'good doctor', they mean a doctor whom they feel they can trust without having to think about it. They equate 'goodness' with integrity, safety, up-to-date medical knowledge and diagnostic skill, and the ability to form a good relationship with them. For them, good doctors are clinically expert and at the same time interested in them, kind, courteous, empathetic and caring.[57]

Patients and doctors are on the same page on this issue.

A broader perspective

My focus so far has been on the qualities an individual patient wants from his or her own doctor, and how that is mirrored in what doctors expect of themselves and fellow doctors. However, society's expectations of doctors are changing. Funders of health care have a keen interest in how effectively doctors serve a whole patient population. Payment mechanisms in primary care are changing from payment on a fee-for-service basis to payment on a capitation basis, where general practitioners are paid an annual amount to care for their enrolled patients. Quality improvement agencies speak of the need to act for the individual patient but think for the population as a whole. Even regulators now emphasise that doctors must think beyond the single patient in front of them. The New Zealand Medical Council is clear about the balancing act required: 'Doctors have a responsibility to the community at large to foster the proper use of resources and must balance their duty of care to each patient with their duty of care to the population. In particular this involves making efforts to use resources efficiently, consistent with good patient care.'[58]

In the United States, healthcare leaders are calling for recognition of the implications of 'the revolution in healthcare delivery', from 'cottage industry to postindustrial care'.[59] In the past, good doctors have been 'celebrated for their unwavering dedication to doing whatever it takes to care for their individual patients … a stereotypical good doctor was independent and always available, had encyclopedic knowledge, and was a master of rescue care'.[60] However, the explosion of medical knowledge, the changing needs of a diverse, ageing patient population, and the complex nature of modern healthcare systems demand a reformulation of what it means to be a good doctor.

Writers in the *New England Journal of Medicine* lay down this challenge: 'Today, a good doctor must have a solid fund of knowledge and sound decision-making skills but also must be emotionally intelligent, a team player, able to obtain information from colleagues and technological sources, embrace quality improvement as well as public reporting, and reliably deliver evidence-based care, using scientifically informed guidelines in a personal, compassionate, patient-centered manner.'[61] We might quibble about aspects of this description, which reads like the job specification for a new age SuperDoctor, but it nicely makes the point that societal and professional expectations are changing our conception of what it means to be a competent doctor in a twenty-first-century health system.

One final observation is necessary. It is not just doctors who are being required to change. Patients are also changing. The model of the passive patient who meekly follows the doctor's orders is being replaced by the patient as an active partner in a therapeutic relationship. Health policy literature now proclaims 'the autonomous patient'. Bioethicist Robert Veatch observes that the 'new medicine' is putting the patient in charge.[62]

These developments are in part a response to consumerism and its impact on healthcare delivery, but also to the growing burden of chronic disease and the inability of doctors acting in traditional roles to meet all their patients' needs. There is also some evidence that better-informed patients have better health outcomes, consume fewer resources (since well-informed patients may opt for non-intervention), and require less time in the long run (if things have been well explained early on).[63]

New models of healthcare delivery are emerging, based on shared decision-making between patients and doctors, with patients bringing their knowledge, values and preferences to the equation, alongside the doctor's expertise.[64] This will require improved health literacy in the general population, and greater availability of decision aids for patients. Increasingly, patients are being encouraged to take responsibility for their own health and therapy. People with a chronic condition are being recognised as 'expert patients' and the idea of 'co-creating' health (supporting people with long-term conditions to develop knowledge, skills and confidence in managing their own health) is gaining currency.[65] Some of these developments may be passing fads. Not all patients have the energy or resources to manage their own health, and it may be unfair to expect them to do so. However, the trend to greater patient engagement is clearly impacting on the role doctors play.

So, a broader perspective on twenty-first-century doctors and patients highlights the importance of communication skills, teamwork, and a commitment to quality improvement in the modern doctor – qualities that complement the more traditional attributes of competence and compassion. We need this broad array of qualities in a good doctor.

Excellence, goodness and badness

A discussion of good doctors and patient expectations can easily lead to a list of aspirational qualities to be aimed for, but unlikely to be found save in occasional paragons of virtue. Professional codes and guidelines are replete with statements about aiming for excellence, and it is natural to think that, if we set the bar higher, we can raise standards across the board.

Let me state my own view. By the good doctor, I mean the 'good enough' doctor. Within any profession, there will always be outliers: the gifted and the ordinary. I want to know that even the ordinary practitioner meets minimum standards, and is someone whom I, and my family, can safely consult. I take this to be what William Osler meant when he wrote: 'In a well-arranged community, a citizen should feel that he can at any time command the services of a man who has received a fair training in the science and art of medicine, into whose hands he may commit with safety the lives of those near and dear to him.'[66]

Standards, as opposed to guidance or goals, are intended to set a mandatory level of performance. Inevitably, they will be open to interpretation and some overlay of reasonableness will be required. But they prescribe a minimum, the floor below which no one should drop. There is an interesting parallel in New Zealand's Code of Health and Disability

Services Consumers' Rights. Right 4(2) of the Code states: 'Every consumer has the right to have services provided that comply with legal, professional, ethical, and other relevant standards.' So if we envisage a standard for good medical practice, it needs to be set at a level that reflects the bottom-line expectations of patients, but not so ambitious as to be beyond the reach of ordinary doctors.

The opposite of a good doctor is generally assumed to be a bad doctor. Yet the same duality of motivation and performance pertains here. Before we ascribe 'badness' to a doctor, we should look for evidence both of motivation to act in a way that harms patients or is indifferent to their welfare, *and* substandard performance. Since the vast majority of doctors are well motivated to care for their patients, their shortcomings are likely to be confined to performance failures. They are not 'bad' doctors, but they are poorly performing and are not 'good enough' to meet patient and professional expectations. I call them 'problem doctors'.

Unfortunately, debate about ensuring that all doctors are good doctors has been bedevilled by the assumption that the task is to weed out 'bad apples'. This negative focus alienates the medical profession, whose cooperation is needed for any system of ensuring good medical practice to be workable. If the task is reconceptualised as ensuring that doctors are 'good enough', the focus can shift to developing clear and attainable standards against which performance can be measured. An individual doctor who does not meet such a standard by definition has not demonstrated 'good enough' practice. There would need to be an opportunity for such a practitioner to remedy the relevant deficiencies and be re-tested against the standard.

Patients do not expect the moon. Indeed, as I will show in Part 2, they often settle for a standard of care, information, and caring that is less than adequate, and does not justify the trust they place in their doctor. The community does not expect excellence, but people do expect to be protected from badness and should be assured that any doctor who cares for them will be a good (enough) doctor.

Assuredly good doctors

Let us assume that most doctors are indeed good (enough) doctors, who exhibit the qualities described above, and are capable of satisfying an assessment against good medical practice standards. Is that an acceptable state of affairs?

I think it is less than ideal. It still leaves a minority of perhaps 5 per cent of doctors who are subpar, including a very small group who are potentially dangerous and unfit to practise. As members of the public, we have few ways – beyond personal experience, the opinions of others and, rarely, published data or decisions – of knowing who are the poorly performing doctors. We are completely reliant on official bodies – principally the medical boards that register doctors and issue annual practising certificates, but also doctors' employers and professional colleges, and agencies handling medical complaints and discipline – to share relevant information and check that every doctor meets appropriate standards.

In an ideal world, we would know that every licensed doctor is a competent doctor – that he or she meets the minimum standards of being a good doctor. The health and regulatory systems would provide us with that assurance. As a member of the public, and a potential patient, I should be able to rely on the fact that someone is listed on the public medical register and has a current licence to practise medicine as assurance that doctor is competent. I do not want to take 'pot luck'. I find it unacceptable that, within the medical community, it is often common knowledge that a certain doctor should be avoided for the care of one's own family, but that the general public is not privy to such information.

In his influential 2006 report *Good Doctors, Safer Patients*, Liam Donaldson, then Chief Medical Officer of England, observed: 'Most doctors know of another doctor whom, on balance, they would prefer not to treat their own family.'[67] Donaldson also noted a 'significant regulatory gap' endangering patient safety: 'Some doctors fall between these two stools, being judged as not "bad enough" for action by the regulator, yet not "good enough" for patients and professional colleagues in a local service to have confidence in them.'[68] This gap must be closed.

I recall being present at a safety and quality meeting in England in 2005 when a Californian health policy expert was asked how we will know we have reached the promised land of safe, patient-centred care. 'When physicians are willing to accept random allocation of a physician for their own and their family's medical care,' he replied.[69]

2
PROBLEM DOCTORS PART OF THE REALITY

In this second part of the book, I shift my focus from the ideal to the reality, in which patients cannot be assured that every licensed doctor is a 'good enough' doctor, and some patients are exposed to harm from 'problem doctors'. I start with a case study, involving an investigation triggered by a family's complaint about the care an elderly general practitioner provided to a trusting, long-time patient. It is a case of 'ordinary failure'. I discuss responsibility for the substandard care.

Moving from the particular to the general, I elaborate on what I mean by problem doctors. I describe some of the scandals and inquiries that have brought this issue to public prominence. Returning to my theme of patient expectations, I examine some of the different ways in which such doctors fall short: by leaving patients in the dark; by exploiting patients; by harming patients; and by treating patients callously. This part of the reality looks rather different from the ideal.

Complaints

Complaints are a good place to start when talking about problem doctors, since they are often how problems come to light. Despite perceptions of the 'public's hue and cry',[1] most patients on the receiving end of poor medical care choose not to make a complaint. Marie Bismark, in her 2006 study looking at the crossover between a sample of patients who suffered an injury from an 'adverse event' in a New Zealand public hospital, and patients from that group who made a complaint to the Health and Disability Commissioner (HDC), found that only 1 in 200 chose to make an official complaint. Even in more serious cases, involving death or disability, only 1 in 25 injured patients complained to HDC.[2] Patients who are elderly or socio-economically deprived are less likely to complain.

The same pattern of under-complaining is likely to occur in general practice, where most patients receive their medical care. The simple fact is that in health care, as in other walks of life, it takes a motivated person to pursue a complaint. You may need all your energy to tackle the health problem you are dealing with. You may feel embarrassed about raising concerns that involve highly personal health issues. You may find it too awkward to complain about your doctor, if he or she is someone you've consulted for a long time.

The fact that most people don't complain is occasionally cited by doctors to suggest that the patients who *do* complain are 'difficult' or whingers. Indeed, a remarkable 31.5 per cent of 598 doctors responding to a survey in 2004 disagreed with the statement that 'complainants are normal people'![3] It is certainly true that the 'norm' is for patients not to complain when their expectations are not met. Obviously that doesn't mean that complainants themselves are abnormal. But it is all too easy to marginalise complainants as a group.

In addition, some commentators assume that because only a small minority of complaints are technically upheld in a formal ruling,[4] that undermines the significance of complaints. This view is wrong on two counts. First, the fact that a patient has been unhappy enough to make a complaint suggests that, from their perspective, something has gone awry and cannot simply be dismissed as irrelevant, even if an objective adjudicator detects no breach of standards. Secondly, although complaints do not require proof of actual harm to a patient (unlike a civil claim for damages for negligence), research indicates that often something *has* gone wrong in the delivery of care. The Bismark study found that in 50 per cent of the complaints to HDC, review of the clinical records showed that there had been an adverse event. The probability of a complaint increases steeply with severity of injury, and preventable events are much more likely to lead to a complaint than unpreventable ones. Thus, complaints offer 'a valuable portal for observing threats to patient safety'.[5]

It always seemed to me that if someone had gone to the trouble of lodging a complaint, there was a question mark over the quality of care or information they had received, and there needed to be a careful assessment of what had happened. I was conscious that complaints are sometimes the tip of the iceberg, a warning of systemic problems in the health system. Even a single complaint about an individual practitioner could be the canary in the coal mine, a sign of an underlying problem that risked harm to other patients, if unaddressed.

An 'ordinary failure'

Naturally, with the passage of time, many of the complaints I handled as Commissioner are dim memories. Only a minority, around 50 a year, led to formal investigations where the results were publicly notified. Over ten years that equates to 500 investigation reports. Some were major inquiries that resulted in a lot of media publicity, remedial changes and, in a few cases, disciplinary or civil proceedings. One particular case sticks in my mind. It involved an elderly general practitioner in the suburbs, and his loyal patient. It never came to media attention and did not lead to public scandal. It was a private scandal, an 'ordinary failure' in a doctor's care for a patient.[6]

The elderly doctor

Dr B was in his mid-seventies and had been in general practice for nearly 50 years. Although his patients probably called him their GP, he was not vocationally registered as a general practitioner; he was registered only in a general scope of registration, and was required to be in a 'collegial relationship' with a vocationally registered GP.

By 2002, Dr B was in semi-retirement working three half-days a week for a suburban medical centre, as an independent contractor paid on a fee-for-service basis. He was described by a colleague as 'a humble and careful man with a deep concern for his patients'. When Dr B joined the practice in 2001, he was reluctant to change his lifelong practice of keeping handwritten notes of his consultations. He had no prior experience of computers, and although he learned to navigate the system, the input of notes into the computer required typing which 'on a part-time basis he did not feel worth learning'. He therefore did not enter patient information in the practice's computerised system, but he could access electronic records on his desk computer, and his colleagues knew to check the manual records if seeing one of Dr B's patients.

The loyal patient
Ms A, aged 62, had been a patient of Dr B for over 20 years. She had multiple pre-existing conditions. In January 2002, Ms A consulted Dr B complaining of dysuria and tenderness high in her abdomen, front and back, and kidney area. Over the next five months, Ms A consulted Dr B on five more occasions with urinary and abdominal symptoms, until he discovered that she had a pelvic cyst. His handwritten records noted only one physical examination, although he claimed to have undertaken three. He initially diagnosed 'urethral irritation' due to sexual activity, and prescribed medication. When her symptoms did not resolve, he prescribed further medication at three consultations, and twice more in response to telephone requests. Dr B did not record his working diagnoses, and did not document any test requests or results.

An ultrasound scan and gynaecological review confirmed the presence of a large pelvic mass 'the size of a 24-week pregnancy'. By August 2002, Ms A had been hospitalised with an ischaemic right leg and, following a CT scan, was found to have cancer of the uterus. Ms A's leg was amputated. She suffered a stroke while in a rehabilitation unit, and died of inoperable cancer several weeks later.

The complaint
Ms A's sister complained to HDC that Dr B had failed to diagnose Ms A's cancer, and that his care had been substandard. An independent expert general practitioner advised HDC: 'Dr B's care was deficient due to his failure to adequately examine and investigate Ms A's urinary and abdominal symptoms' (although the outcome would probably not have

been different) and his notes were 'inadequate in content with Ms A's symptoms poorly recorded, examination findings lacking and management plans deficient'.

As Commissioner, I upheld the complaint and ruled that Dr B had breached his patient's rights by not meeting the legal standard of 'reasonable care and skill' in his management of Ms A, and falling well below professional standards in his record-keeping. The decision was published on the HDC website.[7] I recommended that the New Zealand Medical Council review Dr B's competence and consider whether any conditions should be imposed on his intended occasional future practice (having retired from general practice).

Who was responsible?
Obviously Dr B himself bore a large measure of personal responsibility for his own failings. Dr B's lawyer submitted that the complaint and subsequent proceedings had had a devastating impact on the doctor and had affected his health. Naturally, it is hard to be unmoved by the plight of a doctor who, in the twilight years of his practice, endures an official investigation because of lapses in his care for a single patient. Yet patients are entitled to good care, and proper records, irrespective of the age and experience of their doctor. There can be no sliding standard of care depending on the reputation and seniority of the practitioner. Dr B was personally responsible for failing to maintain his professional competence.

But Dr B was not a sole agent. What responsibility did the medical centre have for Dr B's poor care and records? In its own submission, very little: '[We] have no knowledge of any steps usually taken by medical centres to ensure that locums or doctors are competent other than informal inquiry with their peers and casual overview of their notes at work. Dr B has been in practice for 50 years without a complaint.... We did not "audit" his notes. It did not occur to us to take steps to satisfy ourselves that he was competent.... [T]his is the job of the regulatory authorities.'[8] Dr B's colleagues did not see themselves as their brother's keeper.

What responsibility did the 'regulatory authority' (the New Zealand Medical Council) bear in this situation? The Council's role was not investigated; it is not subject to the jurisdiction of the Commissioner, since it is not a provider of health services. But there was no evidence the Medical Council had taken any steps to check Dr B's ongoing competence, nor that it had any rigorous system in place to do so.

Lessons

What lessons can we learn from this case? I draw the following lessons. Ms A had to take pot luck in seeking medical care. She had no way of knowing whether Dr B was doing his job properly. Like most members of the public who do not have family connections with the medical community, she had to take it on trust that Dr B was competent. As his patient for over 20 years, her trust was long-standing. If asked, she would probably have said, 'Well, he's a professional.' Ms A would have assumed that he needed a 'warrant of fitness' to keep practising. She would have expected his practice colleagues to keep an eye on him, and that the official bodies (the Medical Council) would require him to meet strict practice standards. She was wrong. Her trust was misplaced. When Ms A really needed Dr B to be on the ball, his rusty skills failed him – and her.

I started to wonder how many Dr Bs were practising in New Zealand, and whether anyone was checking. How many problem doctors might there be, and what did it mean for patients?

The problem of problem doctors

The phrase 'problem doctor' is useful shorthand for a fluctuating minority of doctors whose practice of medicine poses a risk to patients. Sometimes, the risk eventuates and patients are harmed. When exposed, such cases lead to public concern and loss of confidence in the medical profession. With some justification, patients, families and the media ask: 'Why wasn't preventive action taken when people knew there was a problem?' Even if no harm results from the doctor's failings, questions arise as to why no one was checking to ensure that standards of good medical practice were being maintained.

To call such doctors 'problem doctors' is apt: they have problems, they pose a risk of harm to patients, and dealing with them is a complex issue for their colleagues, employers and regulatory bodies. It is a catchy phrase, but also a loaded one. To speak of a 'problem doctor' suggests that the doctor *is* the problem, rather than *has* a problem. It is thus likely to alienate many doctors, with its connotations of finger-pointing and scapegoating. They may instinctively empathise with the plight of their fellow practitioner. Doctors may also think: 'There but for the grace of God, go I.'

Some in the medical profession deny that the problem doctor is a major issue, or seek to downplay its significance, compared with systemic factors. Doctors who take this approach mirror the denial frequently exhibited by the doctor with the problem. But many doctors know firsthand, and will concede privately, that it is a difficult and intractable issue. They include leading contemporary American and British medical commentators Atul Gawande and Richard Smith.

Gawande writes: '[D]octors become ill, old, and disaffected or distracted by their own difficulties, and . . . they falter in their care of patients. We'd all like to think of "problem doctors" as aberrations. The aberration may be a doctor who makes it through a forty-year career without at least a troubled year or two. . . . [A]t any given time, an estimated three to five per cent of practicing physicians are actually unfit to see patients.'[9] In a similar vein, Smith comments: 'We shouldn't be surprised by problem doctors. Why wouldn't they exist? Think how surprised we would be by a community . . . where nobody committed terrible crimes, went mad, abused drugs, slacked on the job, became corrupt, lost confidence and competence, or exploited their position.'[10]

Books have been written on this topic, notably two works in the 1990s, *Problem Doctors: A conspiracy of silence*[11] (a collection of essays, mainly by European authors) and *The Incompetent Doctor: Behind closed doors*,[12] in which Marilynn Rosenthal presents her ground-breaking findings from research on doctors in the United Kingdom and Sweden. As the subtitles suggest, a common theme of this literature is that problem doctors exist but their failings are addressed (if at all) in secret. Often it is only when a serious mistake is made, or a patient or family is prompted to make an official complaint, that action is taken.

Although well recognised, the problem of problem doctors endures and elicits inconsistent responses from medical colleagues. In 2009 survey results from 1891 medical specialists in the United States, and 1078 medical specialists in the United Kingdom, 60 per cent of doctors in both countries agreed with the statement that in all instances significantly impaired or incompetent colleagues should be reported to relevant authorities.[13] Nearly 20 per cent of respondents had experience of an impaired or incompetent colleague in the previous three years, and over two thirds had reported the colleague to a relevant authority. The most common action taken by a US physician with knowledge of a problem doctor was to stop referring patients to that doctor (72.4%) – an action much less commonly reported by UK doctors (17.2%). No doubt there would be cultural differences in Australia and New Zealand, but in my experience both countries have a rump of problem doctors whose failings are similarly not always followed up.

The most infamous problem doctors are the ones whose acts and omissions lead to patient deaths, public outcry and official inquiries. In the next section, I consider three major scandals and inquiries, from England, Australia and New Zealand.

Scandals and inquiries

The three cases described in this section are very different, but they illustrate how far some doctors fall from good medical practice, and the limited checks in place to ensure patient safety. Each case demonstrates eloquently and painfully that professionalism is not sufficient on its own to ensure that patients receive care of an appropriate standard, and that external regulation is a necessary part of the equation.

The wrongdoing of Dr Harold Shipman, a general practitioner in Hyde, Manchester, and Dr Jayant Patel, a surgeon in Bundaberg, Queensland, became the focus of highly publicised inquiries. They were convicted respectively of the crimes of murder and manslaughter as a result of patient deaths, so their errant behaviour was obviously highly atypical. Both practitioners were far removed from the good doctors who are the focus of this book. Yet the inquiries into their conduct – and how they were able to harm so many patients – made far-reaching recommendations to protect the public from problem doctors, and led to major reforms of medical regulation in the United Kingdom and Australia.

The third inquiry was triggered by the inadequate review of cytology slides by Dr Michael Bottrill, a pathologist in Gisborne, New Zealand. No crimes were committed, but gaping holes were revealed in quality assurance of the National Cervical Screening Programme. The inquiry highlighted how an incompetent doctor could continue in practice unchecked, exposing patients to avoidable harm. The inquiry recommendations led to changes to the screening programme and the regulatory framework for recertification of health practitioners.

The Shipman Inquiry

'Shipman gave the appearance of being a competent doctor. He was enthusiastic about preventive medicine and undertook regular clinical audit. He seemed to be modern and progressive and was well liked by his patients.'[14] So said Dame Janet Smith, after her exhaustive inquiry into

Harold Shipman's practice. Her view was consistent with the opinion of the son of one of Shipman's patients: 'I remember the time that Shipman gave to my Dad. He would come around at the drop of a hat. He was a marvellous GP apart from the fact that he killed my father.'[15]

Harold Shipman was convicted in January 2000 of the murder of fifteen patients over the years 1995 to 1998, and was sentenced to life imprisonment. The subsequent inquiry concluded that between 1975 and 1998, Shipman had killed no fewer than 215 patients, and may have killed as many as 260. He has the odious distinction of being one of the world's most prolific murderers. Shipman's technique was to administer fatal overdoses of morphine to his victims (mainly middle-aged or elderly female patients), sign their death certificate, and forge their medical records to indicate that they had been in poor health.

The motive for Shipman's killing never became clear prior to his death by suicide in his prison cell in January 2004. It seems that Shipman overcame his own pethidine addiction (which had led to his conviction in 1976 of three offences of obtaining a controlled drug by deception and to a warning from the General Medical Council) but replaced it with an addiction to killing patients by administering lethal doses of morphine.

Harold Shipman was a *bad* doctor – one of the tiny minority of doctors who deliberately harm their patients. (Intentional harm by a doctor usually involves sexual assault rather than seeking to kill or maim, which is as rare in medicine as in other walks of life.) It is very difficult to design systems to catch criminals in medicine, or in any other field of human activity where the provider whose services are ill-intentioned is an expert and the consumer is ill-equipped to judge their technical skills. Shipman was apparently technically proficient and followed clinical guidelines in his everyday practice. Clearly, his patients, his practice staff and other health practitioners in Hyde did not detect that he was a dangerous killer.

The Shipman Inquiry is, nevertheless, relevant to a discussion of patient expectations of good doctors because it dramatically illustrates a number of points: the complete trust of patients in their familiar, long-time doctor; the ability of a clever doctor to deceive patients under the guise of a good bedside manner; the inability of most patients to judge whether a procedure (such as the taking of blood or the administration of a medicine) is clinically necessary or appropriate; and the fact that being guideline compliant and competent in routine medical practice can disguise occasional conduct that is aberrant and abhorrent. It is also noteworthy that Shipman was a general practitioner working in the community, unlike many of the hospital-based specialists whose failings lead to major inquiries.

A number of recommendations from Dame Janet Smith's multi-volume inquiry reports seek to reduce the likelihood of such criminal conduct going undetected, including audits of prescribing data, tighter death certification and cremation rules, more robust coronial procedures, and monitoring of patient mortality data. The judge also commented on the prevailing culture within the medical profession, noting that it was 'not done' for a doctor to report suspicions about a colleague to the authorities.[16] This was seen as a vital area for change: 'There can be no room today for the protection of colleagues where the safety and welfare of patients is at issue. I believe that the willingness of one healthcare professional to take responsibility for raising concerns about the conduct, performance or health of another could make a greater potential contribution to patient safety than any other single factor.'[17] I shall return to this issue in discussing roadblocks, in Part 3.

Dame Janet concluded that 'the problems caused by poorly performing doctors are significant'.[18] She challenged the Government and the General Medical Council to come up with a more rigorous system to revalidate doctors, noting: 'If revalidation were to consist of a periodic assessment of a doctor's competence and fitness to practise, it could make a huge contribution to safeguarding the public against the incompetent and the out of date doctor.'[19] The judge doubted whether the system of revalidation proposed by the Council would detect 'another Shipman'.[20]

I vividly recall my own appearance at the Shipman Inquiry in January 2004. The judge convened a seminar of international experts in health complaint systems and medical regulation, seeking to learn whether more effective systems (perhaps underpinned by legally enforceable patients' rights, as in New Zealand) might detect a Shipman. In her final report, the judge did not recommend such a system for the United Kingdom, although she did propose simplified complaint procedures.

My clearest recollection of appearing at the inquiry is of the judge's questions about how the New Zealand Medical Council ensures the competence and fitness to practise of doctors before renewing their annual practising certificate. It is telling that as Health and Disability Commissioner, the country's leading patient advocate, I was unaware of the basis on which doctors were allowed to continue in practice in New Zealand. I recall spending a lunch break during the inquiry checking the Medical Council's website. So far as I could see – and as I later confirmed to be the case – there was no proactive checking of competence, and the requirements for recertification were very light, limited to a practitioner's declaration of having undertaken some continuing professional development. My interest in the topic of this book was sparked.

The Queensland (Patel) Inquiry

Dr Jayant Patel was an Indian-qualified, US-trained surgeon employed as Director of Surgery at Bundaberg Base Hospital, a public hospital in a provincial city in Queensland, from 2003 to 2005. After numerous complaints from staff were brushed aside, it took the efforts of a determined whistle-blowing nurse, a local journalist and a Member of Parliament, to bring concerns about the standard of Patel's surgery to public attention. A disproportionate number of his patients had died or suffered major surgical complications. Patel was vilified in the media as 'Dr Death'. His surgical performance at Bundaberg Hospital and the circumstances of his appointment and continued employment were scrutinised by retired judge Geoffrey Davies QC, in his 2005 *Queensland Public Hospitals Commission of Inquiry Report*.[21]

The Queensland Inquiry highlighted numerous systemic failures, but also Patel's own 'scandalous conduct'[22] and his contribution to a number of patient deaths and surgical complications. The inquiry cited evidence from an independent clinical review that Patel's 'unacceptable level of care' contributed to thirteen patient deaths (including seven or eight where the treatment was 'outlandish' and involved 'absolutely non defendable processes'), may have contributed to four other patient deaths, and was implicated in 31 other cases of surgical complications.[23] His performance was described as 'incompetent' and 'far worse than average or what one might expect by chance'.[24] Patel was convicted in 2010 of the manslaughter of three patients at Bundaberg Hospital, and of causing grievous bodily harm to another patient on whom he performed unnecessary surgery resulting in the removal of healthy bowel.

The scandal of Bundaberg was that Patel's employer (Queensland Health) and the registration authority (the Medical Board of Queensland) did not make the proper inquiries that would have revealed his troubled disciplinary history and practice limitations in the United States; fellow doctors did not take appropriate action as Patel's surgical inadequacies came to light; and hospital management failed to properly investigate the complaints that Patel attracted from early on in his time at Bundaberg.[25] Patel was rewarded and protected as a prodigious worker who performed a high volume of operations. The inquiry findings vividly illustrated the gap between the rhetoric of rigorous credentialling and quality assurance of medical work, and robust regulatory oversight, and the reality of lax processes that allow a substandard but self-assured specialist to cover his tracks and continue to harm patients – particularly when a publicly funded health service is short-staffed and underfunded, and there is community pressure to ensure the viability of a local hospital.

I recall visiting Queensland Health in March 2005, as chair of an independent committee reviewing governance arrangements for the safety and quality of health care in Australia, shortly before the storm around Patel became public. Senior departmental officials spoke confidently about the safeguards in place to keep patients safe in Queensland Health facilities. That confidence soon dissipated as evidence emerged of the scores of patients harmed at Bundaberg and other Queensland hospitals. Although the issues were far broader than the competence of individual doctors (including the assessment of overseas-trained doctors), that emerged as an important part of the jigsaw puzzle. Patients and families who suffered at the hands of Patel were convinced that he should never have been allowed to do major surgery at Bundaberg Hospital. Their belief was vindicated in the Queensland Inquiry.

Predictably, the Queensland Inquiry led to a complete overhaul of the governance of safety and quality within Queensland Health. It was also an important catalyst for state reforms in Queensland and New South Wales to mandate the reporting of concerns held by one health practitioner about the competence of another practitioner; and precipitated reforms of national health practitioner regulation across Australia, including the creation of the Medical Board of Australia and introduction of mandatory reporting of competence concerns in all states and territories.

One lesson from the Queensland and Shipman inquiries is that it often takes a public scandal and a judicial inquiry to force governments to act, but even then the mood for tougher regulation abates over time, and implementation of reforms in practice often runs into implacable opposition from professional groups wedded to the principle of self-regulation.

Gisborne Cervical Screening (Bottrill) Inquiry

Dr Michael Bottrill worked as the sole permanent pathologist employed by a private laboratory in Gisborne, a provincial city in New Zealand, from 1974 until his retirement in 1996. He was trained in anatomical pathology, not cytopathology. Bottrill became a member of the Royal Australasian College of Pathologists in 1973, after sitting an oral and two practical tests, rather than the full examination. He was admitted under an historic 'grandfather' clause that gave weight to experience over formal qualifications.

Bottrill had no specialist training in cytoscreening, yet from 1990 to 1996 he operated as the sole primary screener reading cervical smears at his private laboratory, and no one checked his work. He attended conferences and meetings in cytology until 1992, but did not 'gain any insight into the risk he was taking by practising as a sole practitioner in cervical cytology, nor ... improve his reading of cervical smear tests'.[26]

One of his patients, Patient A, was diagnosed with cervical cancer requiring radical treatment. She arranged for four of her earlier smears (which had been read by Bottrill) to be re-read; they were found to have been misread. In 1999, as a result of the publicity surrounding Patient A's claim for exemplary damages for negligence,[27] it emerged that some of Bottrill's other patients had also developed cervical cancer following misread smears. Public concern triggered investigations by health authorities and a ministerial inquiry.

A massive re-read of cervical smears (originally read by Bottrill) from over 12,000 women showed that 1997 women had misread smears (including 616 cases involving high-grade abnormalities). Nine deaths from cervical cancer and over 60 cases of alleged injury were revealed in the Gisborne region. The Gisborne Inquiry found serious problems in the running of the National Cervical Screening Programme, noting that '[a]n effective, well-designed and well-implemented programme would have prevented [Bottrill] from practising in this way'.[28]

The Gisborne Inquiry singled out for criticism the fact that Bottrill was able to continue in specialist medical practice for so many years, with no reassessment of his competence:

> There were no compulsory requirements for medical practitioners to undertake formal continuing education, or for them to have their competence reassessed. The Committee considers that this too was a

factor that is likely to have led to the unacceptable under-reporting in the Gisborne region. Had Dr Bottrill been required to undergo formal continuing education and a re-assessment of his competency as a medical practitioner it is unlikely that he would have continued to practice as he did.[29]

Criticism in the inquiry report of the key professional group, the Royal Australasian College of Pathologists, was muted. The storyline from the inquiry was of a flawed system, in which Ministry officials and funding agencies were the villains, rather than the ailing doctor or his professional colleagues. As a result of the inquiry, important changes were made to quality assurance of the Cervical Screening Programme, but (as I will show in Part 4) competence assurance of individual medical practitioners remains a work in progress.

Turning from this trio of high-profile medical scandals and inquiries, what do we know about the types of problem encountered by patients in searching for a good doctor and in receiving medical care? In what ways do patients' everyday experiences sometimes fall short of the ideal of the good doctor?

Problem one: patients in the dark

The lack of information about how to find a good doctor, to judge the quality of one's medical care and, more generally, to choose an appropriate treatment option, is a surprising aspect of being an Antipodean patient in the early twenty-first century. The information abyss is particularly striking in New Zealand, which prides itself on promoting full information disclosure to patients, and where the principle of informed consent has possibly received greater emphasis than in other similar jurisdictions.[30]

New Zealand was one of the first countries in the world to pass a law requiring doctors, nurses and other health practitioners (and all types of providers of health or disability services) to provide patients with information about their condition and treatment options, including the risks, side effects, benefits and costs of each option. The law provides a partial definition of 'informed consent',[31] and numerous decisions from the Health and Disability Commissioner, the disciplinary tribunal, and (to a lesser extent) the courts on appeal have clarified how much information a patient is legally entitled to be given, without asking.[32] These developments can be traced to the 1987–88 Cartwright Inquiry, whose central message was an affirmation of patient autonomy and of the right of patients to receive the information they need to understand their condition and make an informed decision about treatment, and to have that decision respected.

Much progress has been made in giving information to patients in the two decades since the Cartwright Inquiry. But in several important ways, patients in New Zealand remain in the dark. The first, most obvious, knowledge gap is when we want to find a good doctor. Patients looking for a general practitioner or a medical specialist have no easy way to do so. They are likely to turn to the white pages of the telephone book or seek a recommendation from a friend or a doctor or other health practitioner personally known to them. It is difficult enough to find out who is practising in a local area, and whether they are accepting bookings. Reliable information about the quality of doctors is virtually impossible to find. Whatever one might think of the merits of such an idea, there is no publicly available rating of doctors (or, for that matter, other health practitioners, medical centres, rest homes or hospitals). Once again, one is left to rely on personal recommendations.

The lack of reliable comparative information about doctors is remarkable given that we live in the age of consumer demand and readily accessible information, with copious information about products and services available on the internet. The information gap is even more startling in light of the contemporary fixation on health and wellbeing. We can access well-referenced information about symptoms and diseases (as well as much dubious information) online, and this has significant implications for the patient–doctor relationship.[33] Yet patients struggle to find any information about local doctors. Consumer websites such as 'I want great care' (www.iwantgreatcare.org) in the United Kingdom and 'Rate my doctor' in Canada and the United States (www.ratemds.com) have no equivalent in New Zealand or Australia. Survey evidence suggests that many North American consumers want access to information about the quality of care a doctor provides, before seeing a new doctor, whereas fewer New Zealand and Australian consumers have such expectations.[34] The lower expectations of Antipodean consumers may reflect complacency or acceptance of the current information abyss.

The district health boards who employ or fund doctors in the New Zealand public system make no comparative quality information about them available to their communities; the Health and Disability Commissioner declines to name doctors found, on investigation of a complaint, to have provided substandard care; the Ombudsmen responsible for ensuring that public agencies make information publicly available (subject to limited exceptions) support non-disclosure on privacy grounds; and the Medical Council provides sparse information about a doctor's date of graduation, practice district, scope of practice, and conditions (if any) on practice, and whether he or she holds a current practising certificate. (The Council's website is difficult to navigate, as I discovered when undertaking a test search for my own medical brother, despite knowing his district and vocational scope of practice.)

As I will discuss further in Part 4, information about a doctor's track record – for example, rate of complications for a specific procedure, the outcomes of employer credentialling processes or Medical Council competence reviews, and complaints, disciplinary and claims history – is impossible to obtain. (I am not here debating the merits of disclosure, but simply noting the lack of publicly available information.) A 'veil of secrecy' shrouds a lot of information that would be meaningful to patients. There are a few exceptions: where the doctor is one of the handful named by the disciplinary tribunal after a disciplinary offence (which is more likely to relate to unethical conduct or misuse of drugs than to professional negligence), or is named in the media by an aggrieved patient or family. Such information may be useful (we would probably try to avoid a doctor found guilty of exploitative conduct), but it usually relates only to a single event, rather than a pattern of practice, and is unlikely to tell us much about the doctor's competence.

The lack of information continues in the consultation room and in hospital. Informed consent works tolerably well for patients having an anaesthetic and surgery, although it tends to be a document-driven process and often gives patients insufficient time to weigh their options, especially if they are already being primed for theatre. But patients don't just need information before an operation. They need it before all sorts of other healthcare interventions (blood tests, biopsies, X-rays, the prescription of new medicines, referrals to a specialist, etc.), and they need to be told what's going to happen next after their procedure.

All too often, patients are left in the dark. Surveys show that around 20 per cent of New Zealand patients report leaving a general practice consultation with important questions unanswered.[35] They commonly do not know when or whether they will get the results of tests and procedures, and do not receive their results or have them clearly explained.[36] For patients being referred from general practice to a specialist or to hospital, there is frequently a lack of information about when they will be seen and what will happen next. Patients seen in a hospital outpatient clinic, or admitted as an inpatient, often have no idea who their responsible clinician is, and what (if any) plan there is for their course of treatment. For all the talk about care co-ordination, and despite its recognition as a legal right in New Zealand,[37] many patients experience a lack of co-ordination and discontinuity of care.

Doctors would probably accept my claims about the lack of readily accessible information about patients waiting for secondary care services, or in the hospital system, since they themselves often find it difficult to get information about patients they have referred, or who have been discharged to their care. However, some medics contest the claim that patients are given insufficient information. The editor of the *New Zealand Medical Journal* claims that the law requires surgeons to 'do less, talk more and write it all down',[38] and the fact that patients often forget (after surgery) preoperative information is cited as evidence of the futility of informed consent.[39]

As for patients getting information about an individual doctor's track record, many doctors dispute the relevance of such information (arguing that the system or context of care is more important than the individual practitioner), invoke their personal privacy interests, and warn that moves to greater information disclosure would cause some doctors to abandon practice, making it more difficult for patients to access medical care. These are contentious issues, but the relative paucity of information available to New Zealand patients is an observable fact.

Problem two: the exploitation of patients

The second problem – the exploitation of patients by doctors – occurs rarely. When such conduct is proven, it usually leads to professional discipline and practice limitations. Despite the rarity of such cases, when they do occur they highlight the peculiar vulnerability of patients.

Patients are vulnerable to sexual, financial and other forms of exploitation by doctors, given the physical and psychological intimacy of the patient–doctor relationship. It is often categorised as a fiduciary relationship in which the patient reposes trust and confidence in the doctor. Although academics debate whether such a characterisation is legally accurate,[40] it is clear that doctors are subject to well-recognised fiduciary obligations, including a duty of confidentiality and a duty not to exploit their patient.

The right to be free from 'sexual, financial or other exploitation' is affirmed in right 2 of New Zealand's Code of Consumers' Rights, with 'exploitation' defined to include 'any abuse of a position of trust, breach of a fiduciary duty, or exercise of undue influence'.[41] The practice of medicine gives doctors legitimate access to a patient's body and, in the private system, to his or her wallet. Both entrées can open the door to unscrupulous conduct by a deviant doctor.

Sexual misconduct towards a patient is the most common reason doctors are disciplined in New Zealand and Australia (being the primary issue in around one quarter of cases resulting in discipline), but it is still very rare, given that only 6 out of 10,000 doctors annually are found guilty of any form of misconduct by a disciplinary tribunal.[42] Furthermore, two thirds of sexual misconduct cases involve sexual relationships with patients, as opposed to other forms of inappropriate sexual contact.[43] The rate of sexual exploitation by doctors, at least based on reported cases that lead to discipline, is therefore extremely low.

Within this rare category of breach of trust, two types of sexual misconduct are clearly exploitative. The first is the egregious situation where a doctor sexually assaults a patient. Because of the extraordinary breach of trust in such cases, there is invariably widespread publicity and condemnation when the offending doctor is brought to justice. Examples in recent years include, from England, psychiatrists William Kerr (convicted of indecent assault on a patient) and Michael Haslam (convicted of four counts of indecent assault on a patient); and from New Zealand, general practitioner Morgan Fahey (convicted of rape of one female patient, sexual violation of another, and indecent assault on eleven patients). The inquiries into these doctors' offending highlighted a long-standing pattern of inappropriate behaviour and that patients faced barriers in seeking to pursue an allegation of sexual assault against their doctor. Serious offending was able to continue unchecked despite clear warning signs.

Sexual misconduct that is not criminal may also be exploitative. The New Zealand Medical Council has taken a strong stance in its official guidance, *Sexual Boundaries in the Doctor–Patient Relationship: A resource for doctors*, adopting a so-called 'zero tolerance' policy. The Council describes any form of sexual behaviour with a current patient as an 'abuse of trust'.[44] In contrast to the regulator's firm line, disciplinary tribunals and the courts are sometimes reluctant to discipline doctors who enter into consensual intimate relationships with patients who are not psychologically vulnerable, describing the doctor's behaviour as unethical or unwise rather than exploitative.[45] However, there are many examples of sexual behaviour that, while technically consensual, is highly exploitative – for example, the psychiatrist who enters into a sexual relationship with a sexually abused woman he is treating. In these cases, courts and disciplinary tribunals are rightly condemnatory.[46]

Cases of direct financial exploitation occur in medicine, but are relatively uncommon. Such conduct may be defined as where a doctor exploits or takes advantage of his privileged position vis-à-vis the patient to secure personal financial gain. Examples of direct exploitation include the doctor who preys on an elderly patient to secure a loan or bequest. Obviously, doctors have less ready access to a patient's financial affairs than an accountant or lawyer, but an ailing patient who needs frequent medical care and becomes close to his or her doctor may be vulnerable to pleas for financial assistance.

Indirect financial exploitation is more common, but less readily detectable. The practice of modern medicine can be a highly profitable business, and there are numerous opportunities for doctors to seek financial reward in subtle ways that are exploitative of patients. The commercialisation of medicine makes doctors subject to a wide array of financial incentives with the potential to cloud their clinical judgement about the patient's best interests.[47] It is these sorts of pressures, especially but not exclusively in the United States, that have been a key driver behind efforts to reaffirm statements of medical professionalism and commitment to patient welfare and patient autonomy.

Examples abound. They include booking a patient for clinically unnecessary repeat consultations for which the doctor is able to bill on a fee-for-service basis; the surgeon who performs and bills for unnecessary operations; the specialist who refers patients seen in the public system to his private practice without adequate disclosure of the option of publicly funded treatment; the specialist who books patients for assessment and follow-up at his private clinic, when they could receive free consultations in the public system; the doctor who has an undisclosed arrangement with a supplier to prescribe a particular medication or product; and the general practitioner who peddles alternative health products, for which he receives a commission, to patients.

There are other forms of exploitation by doctors of patients, where neither sex nor money is involved. In rare cases, doctors expose patients to harm for their own ends, as occurred in the case discussed below, where a drug-addicted physician at Gisborne Hospital undertook unnecessary colonoscopies, to provide an excuse to prescribe pethidine, which he then used for himself while substituting saline solution for the unknowing patients.[48] Such cases appal doctors as much as the community at large.

More contentious, though in my view still exploitative, are the situations where a doctor undertakes research on a patient during the course of treatment, or uses a patient for teaching purposes, without his or her informed consent. No matter how well intentioned the doctor, such conduct is exploitative of the patient. The Code of Consumers' Rights extends patients' rights to participation in research or teaching, and requires advance notification and consent for such activities.[49]

In New Zealand, the most infamous example was gynaecologist Herbert Green's 'unfortunate experiment' on more than 100 women patients at National Women's Hospital with cervical carcinoma *in situ*, who were monitored but did not receive the standard treatment of cone biopsy, resulting in many cases of invasive cancer. The exploitation of vulnerable, unsuspecting female patients was detailed in Judge Cartwright's *Report* of the Cervical Cancer Inquiry.[50] Other abhorrent practices revealed during the Cartwright Inquiry were also exploitative of patients, including students practising the insertion of intra-uterine devices on anaesthetised women without their consent, and the taking of vaginal smears from newborn babies without parental consent.

With strict requirements now in place for ethical approval and written consent for research in New Zealand, it is very unusual for patients to be unwittingly turned into research or teaching subjects. But from time to time the Health and Disability Commissioner sees examples of such behaviour: the general surgeon who, in the course of gall bladder surgery, took liver biopsy samples without consent for research purposes;[51] and the neurology patient who agreed to be part of a teaching session, but had not understood that it would involve 40 to 60 GPs attending 'the demonstration', and felt humiliated and embarrassed.[52] Good intentions cannot disguise the exploitation in such cases, and it is easy to understand the disbelief that fuels a patient's complaint on learning of the breach of trust.

Problem three: doctors who harm patients

The third situation where problem doctors cause problems for patients is when such doctors harm them. It is important to emphasise that the vast majority of harm caused by doctors is unintentional. Most doctors do not seek to harm their patients, a fact sometimes forgotten by the media when baying for the blood of an errant doctor whose negligent act or omission has killed a patient.

Medical murder
As we have seen, there are exceptions. Harold Shipman was a serial killer who murdered his patients. He was a criminal and a bad doctor. His American counterpart is Michael Swango. Between 1984 and 1997, Swango fatally poisoned up to 60 patients during a medical career that

took him from Illinois to South Dakota, New York and Zimbabwe before the FBI tracked him down and he was found guilty of three murders and sentenced to life imprisonment. Even as a medical student he had been nicknamed 'Double-o Swango – licensed to kill', after five of his patients died mysteriously at Southern Illinois University. There were numerous warning signs throughout his career, notably his conviction in 1985 of aggravated battery for poisoning co-workers, leading to a lengthy prison sentence. Yet Swango managed to start afresh, finding medical work in new locations using forged documents. The gripping story of his trail of killing, and how he evaded state medical boards for so long, is aptly entitled *Blind Eye: How the medical establishment let a doctor get away with murder*.[53]

Assault and other forms of deliberate harm

Harm may be deliberately inflicted in other ways by malevolent medics. Such misconduct is exceedingly rare, but the perpetrators may be able to evade detection for a long time because it is so unthinkable that a trusted doctor would act in this way. Gynaecologist Graeme Reeves, the 'butcher of Bega' in New South Wales, is one recent example. He was found guilty of maliciously inflicting grievous bodily harm on a patient whose genitals he removed without her consent,[54] and of assaulting two patients during pelvic examinations.[55] At the time of writing, anaesthetist James Peters of Melbourne, Victoria is suspected of deliberately infecting patients with hepatitis C at an abortion clinic where he worked. A public health inquiry found that 49 of his patients tested with the same strain of hepatitis C as Dr Peters; Victoria's Chief Health Officer said that it was hard to believe the women had been 'accidentally' infected.[56] Dr Peters has been charged with 54 counts of conduct endangering life, negligently causing serious injury and recklessly causing serious injury.[57]

Medical manslaughter

At the borderline of the criminal law are cases where a doctor's reckless or grossly negligent conduct kills or harms a patient. The criminal code contains several generic provisions that can be applied in such situations. In a series of prosecutions in the 1980s and 1990s, four doctors in New Zealand (two anaesthetists, one surgeon and one radiologist) were convicted of manslaughter as a result of negligent acts or omissions that resulted in a patient's death. Following a highly effective campaign by the Medical Law Reform Group, and a report by retired Court of Appeal judge Sir Duncan McMullin, the law was amended in 1997 to require 'a *major departure* from the standard of care expected of a reasonable person' in such circumstances.[58] In essence, this introduced a requirement of 'gross' rather than 'ordinary' negligence, and greatly reduced the risk of turning 'good people into criminals'.[59]

Since the law change, no doctors have been prosecuted for 'medical manslaughter' in New Zealand, and there seems no realistic prospect of a revival of use of the criminal law in this area. Most patient advocacy groups, doctors and lawyers would now agree that, in healthcare settings, the criminal law should be reserved for cases of deliberate harm or gross negligence – for example, the doctor who is absent without leave when on call, or drunk on duty, or who blindly continues with a risky procedure without proper regard for the consequences. Apart from such cases, it is generally accepted that careless doctors should be held accountable through civil processes, including incident review, performance assessment by a medical board (if there is evidence of a possible underlying competence problem), and a complaint investigation and disciplinary process, if warranted.

Resort to the criminal law may frustrate the regular mechanisms for health professional accountability and cast a chilling shadow over the health sector. It risks driving mistakes underground. Yet, intriguingly, there is renewed interest in the use of the criminal law in relation to grossly negligent doctors in the United Kingdom and Australia. As noted earlier, surgeon Jayant Patel was convicted by a Queensland court of the manslaughter of three patients, and of causing grievous bodily harm to another. The Patel case has highlighted the possibility of 'doctors in the dock' in Australia in exceptional cases.

Reckless harm

One area where reckless behaviour may harm patients is where their doctor continues to practise while in the throes of an untreated addiction to alcohol or drugs.[60] Doctors are at increased risk of addiction to prescription medicines, especially abuse involving opiates and benzodiazepines.[61] The ready access to such medicines provides a partial explanation for drug addiction being a particular problem amongst doctors.

This is a problem well known to medical boards, but largely invisible to the general public. Considerations such as the privacy of the doctor (and their family), the tragedy of addiction, workforce shortages, and the pressure to allow redemption so that an otherwise good doctor can use their skills for public good, mean that rehabilitation is often pursued, despite the risk to patient safety in the event of a relapse.

In addition to the obvious risk of mistakes while under the influence, there is a further, insidious risk in the case of a doctor who is addicted to prescription medicines that are readily available in a hospital setting. The addiction may lead such doctors to self-administer stolen medicines intended for their patients. The extent of deception and harm that can result is well illustrated in the following case from New Zealand

Case study – the doctor addicted to prescription medicines
Dr A was a specialist physician in his forties, working at Gisborne Hospital in New Zealand. A decade earlier, while working in another small hospital, he had become addicted to opiates. He had notified his employer and the Medical Council, and voluntarily withdrawn from practice while undergoing inpatient specialist addiction treatment. In 1996, he entered a voluntary agreement to undergo regular medical

monitoring overseen by the Council. In 1997, with approval from the Council, he resumed practice at Gisborne Hospital, where key management and clinical personnel were informed that he was being monitored for drug addiction. Council's monitoring continued until 2004, when it was considered safe to discontinue it.

In 2005, nurses at Gisborne Hospital noticed a change in Dr A's prescribing practices. He was increasingly prescribing intravenous pethidine for procedures such as sigmoidoscopies. Concerns were raised with hospital management, and after an investigation Dr A was confronted and eventually confessed that he had been prescribing pethidine unnecessarily for patients and instead administering it on himself. This had commenced in 2000, when he was still being monitored. There had been a 'distortion' of his practice, whereby he substituted saline solution for pethidine (especially for patients undergoing sigmoidoscopy); he admitted doing this about 40 to 50 times in 2005.

Dr A resigned from the hospital in 2006, and entered a further voluntary intensive medical monitoring and treatment programme overseen by the Health Committee of the Medical Council. In subsequent disciplinary proceedings, he was found guilty of professional misconduct for improperly prescribing pethidine, using it on himself, and administering saline to patients as a substitute. This was a 'very serious breach' of a doctor's professional obligation to 'do no harm'. At least one patient had a procedure that was not necessary; other patients may have had unnecessary procedures. The disciplinary tribunal was sympathetic to Dr A's efforts to overcome his addiction, but considered that he would always remain an addict, with a real risk of relapse. He was permitted to practise only in a general practice (not as a specialist physician), subject to strict conditions. Dr A was fined $10,000, censured, ordered to pay costs, and named. On appeal to the High Court, the tribunal's order that Dr A be suspended for twelve months, given the seriousness of his offending, was quashed, although the other penalties were upheld (subject to one minor variation).[62]

Negligent harm

By far the largest category of harm caused to patients by doctors involves conduct that is not criminal or reckless, but inadvertent. Most commonly, inadvertent patient harm results from a combination of systemic problems and human error. That does not deter people from pointing the finger at individuals. Patients and their families, and even colleagues and managers, are often quick to assume that a careless practitioner is responsible for an adverse event. It is human nature to blame operator error; the doctor or nurse who gives the wrong medication is obviously the proximate cause, 'but for' which the error would not have occurred. Looked at in isolation, they have acted negligently. But the stage has usually been set for the error by a series of upstream, latent errors that could have averted the harm. Much of the energy of the patient safety movement in recent years has been directed towards addressing these underlying factors and 'fixing' the system.

Several major epidemiological studies have confirmed the prevalence of adverse events in health care. Around 1 in 10 patients in modern health systems suffer iatrogenic (healthcare-induced) harm. Some harm (a patient's unexpected allergy or surgical complications) is an unavoidable side effect of treatment properly given. But around 40 per cent of adverse events are preventable, and included in that significant body of avoidable harm are cases of individual medical negligence.

The common or garden variety of negligence cases occur where a patient is harmed by a doctor's failure to exercise the reasonable care and skill to be expected in the particular circumstances. Injured patients may receive restorative treatment (if feasible) and be able to recover damages for negligence in common law systems (often avoided by settlement payments made by insurance companies on behalf of doctors and their employers) or to claim publicly funded compensation (in countries such as New Zealand and Denmark).

There is now much greater openness in cases of negligent or inadvertent harm. Clinicians and managers have come to realise that where injured patients are not faced with a wall of silence, they may be less likely to pursue legal remedies. The change in approach may be due to self-interest, or to an attitudinal shift within the medical profession, prompted by the emphasis on 'open disclosure' in ethical guidelines and tribunal rulings. Patients are increasingly likely to be told that a mistake has been made, to receive an explanation and apology, and to be given information about the steps being taken to prevent a recurrence of the mistake.

Candour and commitment to improvement should do much to restore trust in doctors and the health system. These forms of redress are consistent with research about patient expectations when making a complaint. Research confirms my own observation from reading hundreds of patient complaints: the majority of complainants are motivated by the altruistic motive of seeking to prevent the same thing happening to someone else (by correction of the underlying problem) and a desire for communication about what happened.[63] The oft-cited 'vexatious' complainant is, in practice, rarely encountered.

Nevertheless, some complainants do want to see an errant doctor punished. I recall the surgeon who oversaw New Zealand's medical complaints system in the 1980s decrying the fact that some complainants sought 'blood on the floor, preferably male, medical and Caucasian'![64] While that claim seems exaggerated, there is evidence that, following an adverse event, a small minority (12%) of injured patients and families seek accountability in the form of sanction of the individual practitioner involved in their care.[65] They may pursue a complaint to an employer, a health ombudsman or a medical board, seeking some or all of practice limitations (including suspension or striking off the register) and professional discipline.

Sanction is more likely to be demanded in cases of repeated substandard care. Even the most altruistic patient is likely to take a dim view of situations where the harm may have been prevented by proper mechanisms to detect and respond to a pattern of substandard medical care. It is no wonder the women of Gisborne, who suffered preventable harm at the hands of incompetent pathologist Michael Bottrill, felt betrayed by the health system that should have protected them.

In Part 3, I discuss the combination of inertia, medical culture, legal barriers and bureaucracy that combine to make inaction all too common a response to the poorly performing practitioner, even in the face of preventable patient harm. In such cases, the reality falls well short of patient expectations of assuredly good doctors.

Problem four: doctors who treat patients callously

The final group of problem doctors (in my idiosyncratic classification) comprises those doctors who treat patients callously. Of course, any doctor can have an 'off day' and act in a brusque or unfeeling way to a patient. An occasional lapse is probably inevitable given the heavy demands on doctors' time. My concern is with doctors who treat patients callously.

I use the phrase 'callous' to describe behaviour that any reasonable bystander would describe as heartless, unkind or uncaring, even if that was not the intention of the doctor. My focus is on the doctor who engages in such behaviour on an ongoing basis – in which case it seems reasonable to describe the conduct as intentional, and the doctor who behaves in this way as a problem doctor.

As noted in Part 1, patients highly value being treated with respect and shown kindness and compassion. Although the latter qualities are desirable, treatment with respect is a bottom line, and a legal entitlement for patients in New Zealand and the United Kingdom.[66] Despite these worthy laws, lack of respect – by keeping patients waiting and putting the needs of providers first – persists as a feature of the New Zealand health system and the National Health Service in the United Kingdom, as in other modern health systems. Callous conduct occurs less often, and is one of the worst forms of disrespect for patients.

I recall the case of the fearful middle-aged woman who consulted a general surgeon about a procedure to confirm whether she had pancreatic cancer, recently diagnosed by her local specialist. The surgeon interrupted the consultation to take a long telephone call about a business matter, and later said that he would be away for a month, commenting: 'If I don't have a holiday, I might die.'[67] The first act was thoughtless, the second grossly insensitive. Together, they amounted to callous behaviour.[68]

When such behaviour occurs on a single occasion, is remedied by an apology, and is not repeated, that should be the end of the matter. Stressed and overworked clinicians can sometimes act in a way that is out of character and forgivable. But where a doctor regularly treats patients callously, he or she merits the description 'problem doctor'.

Another case comes to mind, involving a general surgeon working in a public hospital. He told a morbidly obese female patient in her forties, consulting him about the possibility of bariatric surgery, that she would need to go on a 'fucking diet', after she had described her history of failed diets and her aversion to the word 'diet'. When she wrote to complain, the surgeon offered a quasi-apology but said that he was a straight talker, and that in light of the breakdown in their therapeutic relationship, he was removing her from his waiting list. During my investigation of her complaint, the hospital's Medical Director explained that hospital management tolerated the surgeon's 'foul mouth' (although he had been asked to tone down his language) because he was highly competent. The excuse did not wash; the surgeon's swearing and subsequent retaliation struck me as cruel and callous, and both the surgeon and his employer were held liable for his conduct.[69]

Callous conduct is disturbingly common in the health system. A prime culprit is the 'disruptive doctor', who treats patients with contempt, bullies junior doctors and nurses, and refuses to co-operate with reasonable requests from colleagues and management. Disruptive doctors are becoming recognised as a problem in the health service. Dealing with them takes excessive time and energy, but if left unaddressed they can wreak havoc. The New Zealand Medical Council has followed other regulators in issuing guidance to employers about their responsibility to 'adopt a consistent, proactive "zero tolerance" approach to destructive behaviour'.[70] When an occasional outburst becomes a regular pattern of conduct, intervention is essential to protect patients from the psychological harm of being treated callously or witnessing disruptive behaviour, and from the risk of physical harm from an adverse event triggered by a breakdown in teamwork.

Predictably, there appears to be a correlation between disruptive behaviour and incidents, adverse events and patient complaints. Health inquiries into the harm caused by a poorly performing practitioner will often reveal prior instances of treating patients badly, which in retrospect can be seen as red flags that all was not well. Slovakian-trained gynaecologist Roman Hasil was the subject of a major inquiry in New Zealand, arising out of the high failure rate in tubal ligations he performed at Wanganui Hospital.[71] During my inquiry, allegations were made of callous behaviour towards female patients. Subsequently, Australian medical authorities reopened investigations into allegations of such behaviour during Hasil's previous employment in a New South Wales Hospital. The warning signs had been there all along.

In the absence of a third party witness, complaints about a doctor's cruel remarks often turn into a 'she said, he said' dispute, difficult for fact finders to resolve, and all too easily dismissed as miscommunication. But where a number of patients or colleagues report such behaviour, a firm response by employers and regulators is essential, to prevent harm to patients. Patients do not expect to be treated this way by doctors. They describe such behaviour as 'unprofessional'. To my mind, it is well captured by the quaint phrase in traditional medical practitioner legislation, 'conduct unbecoming a medical practitioner'. Whatever label is applied, the doctor who treats a patient callously falls well short of our expectations of a good doctor.

Preventing harm to patients

The four problems described in this part are very different: patients in the dark; exploitation of patients; doctors who harm patients; and doctors who treat patients callously. The doctors who withhold information from patients, or who unintentionally harm them, may be hapless actors in a complex health system. The doctors who exploit, cause deliberate harm, or treat patients callously are morally blameworthy practitioners, who deserve to be punished.

From a patient perspective, the differences may not be so great. They suffer harm at the hands of their doctor and health system. They will almost certainly lose trust in their doctor. If that is compounded by the failure of colleagues, employers and regulators to respond adequately, they will have diminished trust in the medical profession as a whole. It is no wonder that medical self-regulation is increasingly under threat, and demands for greater accountability are growing.

Much of the harm suffered by patients is preventable, yet problems endure. In Part 3, I examine the roadblocks that have hindered solutions to these problems, and contributed to calls for regulatory reform so that patients can be assured of good doctors. Why is the ideal of good medical practice so difficult to achieve?

3

THE ROADBLOCKS
WHY IS CHANGE SO DIFFICULT?

In this third part of the book, I examine why achieving the ideal, in which patients can be assured that every licensed doctor is a 'good enough' doctor, is so difficult. If patients and doctors largely agree that patient expectations of a good doctor are reasonable, why is there such resistance to the changes necessary to check that standards are being maintained? Why are patients routinely deprived of the information they need to make informed choices? Why does the problem of problem doctors persist? Why does it sometimes take a determined complainant and the involvement of the media to force the hand of reluctant regulators? Is a system of assuredly good doctors destined to remain an unattainable ideal?

The players and the system

To understand the obstacles to change, it helps to identify the key actors and their roles in the health system. Who are the *dramatis personae*? Obviously the central figures are the patients themselves and the doctors who care for them. But there is a significant supporting cast. On the patient side, there will often be family members and friends who support and advocate for them. Sometimes there will be a formal 'patient advocate'.[1] At the macro level, there may be a patient advocacy group promoting the rights of patients in general or the needs of patients with a specific disease or chronic condition.

On the doctor's side, there is a larger cast of characters. There will be practice colleagues: the practice nurse or receptionist, in a small general practice; and the team of doctors, nurses and allied health workers in a hospital. These are the people who work alongside the doctor in caring for the patient. At one remove, other health practitioners may have a broad oversight role: the director of quality in a primary care organisation or the chief medical officer in a hospital. Professional peers also play a part, both as equals practising the same specialty, and as superiors with oversight responsibilities, such as the clinical director of a specialty division within a hospital.

In all but the smallest healthcare organisations, there will be the much-maligned managers, with line management and budgetary responsibilities. When there is a performance problem involving an individual practitioner or team, it will frequently be escalated to the relevant manager. Managers in the health system have power, but their degree of influence is variable and depends on the support of clinicians and senior management. Above the managers, at the top of the hierarchy in most healthcare organisations, there will be a chief executive, who generally reports to a board of directors. The board and CEO will usually be invisible to the patient, but they set the agenda for the organisation (including whether safety and quality or increased profitability is the main goal), and they are rightly held to account for major problems that impact on patient care.

Widening our focus, the funders of health care come into view. In health systems in which public funding predominates (such as in Canada, the United Kingdom, Australia and New Zealand), statutory health authorities will be charged with funding health services to meet the needs of regional populations, subject to detailed eligibility criteria. These authorities enter into contracting arrangements with healthcare organisations, and typically specify defined outputs (e.g., volume of surgical operations to be performed) or outcomes (e.g., vaccination targets to be achieved for a designated population). In health systems such as the United States, where private funding predominates (beyond the large Medicare and Medicaid programmes funded by federal and state governments), employers are the major funders of health care. In all health systems patients are to some extent funders of health care, both indirectly as taxpayers and directly in paying out of pocket for services that are not publicly funded, nor available under any applicable insurance cover.

Ministers of Health, and their policy advisors from within the Ministry or Department of Health, play key roles. Ministers sit at the

Cabinet table and argue the case for more public funding for health care; they have important statutory powers and responsibilities in the health arena; they appoint many of the regulators in the health system; and their head is on the block if a major health scandal erupts on their watch. In the Westminster system of government, Ministers are elected politicians who serve at the pleasure of the Prime Minister and the electorate. In contrast, the Directors-General of Health who advise Health Ministers are usually public servants with expertise in public sector management and health policy. On the legislative side, the Health Select Committee of Parliament acts as an important check on legislative proposals, and may undertake inquiries into aspects of health system performance.

Beyond central government, there is a range of statutory agencies and ministerial advisory committees relevant to good medical practice. Prime examples are bodies that handle complaints and concerns about healthcare providers, or promote patient safety and quality improvement. In New Zealand, Australia and the United Kingdom, healthcare complaint commissioners or health ombudsmen undertake the former role. In most modern health systems, a safety and quality agency (such as the Australian Commission on Safety and Quality in Health Care) has become a standard part of governance arrangements.

Beyond the executive branch of government is the judicial system. The courts come into focus at the point where the health and legal systems intersect. When concerns about a doctor's competence escalate into complaints, employer investigations and official inquiries, the affected doctor may seek recourse to the courts to challenge adverse findings, or even to stop an inquiry in the first place. In such cases, judicial process and the law (including the requirements of natural justice, the rules of evidence and constraints of employment law) may determine the scope and outcome of a competence review. Alternatively, an injured patient or bereaved family may bring a civil claim and face the barriers of the law of negligence in seeking to hold an individual doctor or employing authority liable for damages. Coroners (technically, courts) and disciplinary and administrative tribunals (which have adjudicative functions, but are not courts) also play a role in considering whether poor performance contributed to a patient's death, or merits professional discipline or sanction.

Far more intricately involved in the regulation of health care are the professional regulatory bodies. In former British colonies, like Australia and New Zealand, medical boards have traditionally been modelled on the General Medical Council (GMC) of the United Kingdom, dominated by senior doctors appointed as Council members by the Minister of Health, and headed by a Council President. Canada has a similar model, with provincial bodies known as colleges of physicians and surgeons. In the United States, the equivalent bodies are state medical boards.

The GMC itself has changed dramatically, as a result of governance reforms following the Bristol and Shipman inquiries; an equal number of twelve medical and twelve lay members, and a medical chair, all appointed by an Independent Appointments Commission, form the modern GMC. The Antipodean medical councils continue to be dominated by doctors, with limited lay membership (four out of twelve); members are appointed by the Minister of Health, although in New Zealand the Minister has agreed to reserve four of the eight medical member places for doctors elected by the profession.[2]

The university medical schools where students obtain medical degrees, and the professional colleges that provide postgraduate vocational medical training and certify doctors as specialists of various stripes (surgeons, physicians, psychiatrists, general practitioners, etc.), are important players in the health system. They prepare the medical workforce and determine whether students and trainees learn only clinical knowledge and skills, or develop additional competencies in communication, teamwork and patient safety. Ministries of Health, medical boards and employers rely heavily on professional colleges to confirm that doctors are equipped to undertake specialist roles. The admission of a doctor as a 'Fellow' of a specialty college (traditionally a 'royal' college) is the official seal of approval of their fitness for purpose for a specialist role.

THE ROADBLOCKS

A number of organisations advocate for doctors. Most prominent are the medical professional organisations, known by their acronyms: the AMA (the American Medical Association or the Australian Medical Association), the BMA (the British Medical Association), CMA (the Canadian Medical Association) and the NZMA (the New Zealand Medical Association). Although their membership may fluctuate (around 42% of practising doctors in New Zealand belong to the NZMA),[3] they generally have the ears of Ministers of Health and are the first port of call for journalists covering health news. Their pronouncements on new health policy proposals often get disproportionate coverage in the popular press. They promulgate influential codes of medical ethics. Their mandate includes advocating for patients, but their most forceful advocacy is often on behalf of medical practitioners.

Medical unions (such as the Association of Salaried Medical Specialists and the Resident Doctors' Association in New Zealand) sit alongside medical associations and engage in collective bargaining over conditions of employment for members. They are a significant voice when health regulatory reforms affecting their members are mooted. Also influential are the medical defence organisations, indemnity insurers who provide advice and legal representation for insured members of the medical profession. They are usually engaged when a doctor faces a complaint, incident review, coronial inquiry, investigation or disciplinary proceeding. Defence organisations (such as the Medical Protection Society operating in New Zealand and the United Kingdom) seek to ensure that an insured doctor is treated fairly in any legal process, and that the terms of any competence review are carefully circumscribed. They take an intense interest whenever changes are proposed to the medico-legal system.

Last but not least is the media. Stories about individual patients who die or are injured during medical treatment, or who are exploited or mistreated, are grist to the media mill. Where several patients are affected, and allegations emerge of substandard care and lax oversight by health authorities, the result is a potent mix that ensures widespread news coverage and can easily lead to demands for answers from employers, medical boards and Health Ministers, and to calls for an independent inquiry. In the politics of health, the medium is often the message.

As can be seen, there are many players in the health system. All would claim to desire a situation where patients can be assured of finding a 'good enough' doctor by relying on the public medical register. All would deprecate the underbelly of poor practice in the medical profession, though there would be vigorous debate about the extent of the problem. Where the various actors part company is in their assessment of the roadblocks that impede improvement, and in their prescription for change. Let's start with the roadblocks.

Undemanding patients

The demanding patient, who has great expectations of what doctors, nurses and the health system can deliver, is a familiar figure in contemporary debate about health policy. Such patients, it is claimed, make unrealistic demands for futile treatment; expect doctors to spend hours explaining remote risks and far-fetched options; believe that treatment success can be guaranteed; complain noisily when their expectations are not fulfilled; and 'drive' defensive medicine.

It is difficult to find solid evidence to support these claims. True, some families are demanding, and expect doctors and nurses to 'dance to a patient's family tune' and act as if their family member 'was the ward's only patient and that their demands came before the needs of any others'.[4] Some patients have unrealistic expectations of the miracles that modern medicine can perform, make excessive demands for treatment, and become unhappy and complain when their wishes are not complied with. The best efforts of staff cannot satisfy them. Complaint managers and patient liaison officers in hospitals state that there are more 'squeaky wheels' in the system than there used to be, and that they take up a disproportionate amount of time and resources.

It is certainly true that healthcare complaints are rising. Complaints to the Health and Disability Commissioner rose by over 40 per cent in the decade from 2000, and Australasian healthcare complaint commissioners report similar increases. In the UK, the General Medical Council reported a record number of complaints and disciplinary hearings against doctors in 2010.[5]

The increase in complaints is likely attributable to greater consciousness in a consumer society that patients are entitled to complain, and to doctors and their employers being more likely to raise concerns about their medical colleagues. Yet (as noted in Part 2) the vast majority of patients never complain, even when things go wrong. In my experience, despite the rhetoric about demanding patients, it is generally the patients themselves who are subject to expectations: to be patient; not to waste the doctors' and nurses' time; to be grateful for whatever an overstretched health system can deliver; to follow instructions and be compliant; to accept that mistakes happen; and to forgive and not complain when presented with the ritual of 'open disclosure' and systems learning (in other words, when clinicians openly disclose to a patient or family what happened and why, and explain the steps being taken to prevent a recurrence).

Who suffers most in the current system, in which patients cannot be assured of having a good doctor, experience variable standards of care and, in a small minority of cases, are treated by incompetent doctors? The obvious answer is the patients themselves. One might therefore expect patients to be demanding change. But there is little evidence of that. The Consumers Health Forum of Australia and Women's Health Action in New Zealand have lobbied for better regulatory protection for patients. In the United Kingdom, some consumer advocacy groups, such as the Patients Association and the Picker Institute, have been strongly supportive of regulatory reforms to ensure that doctors' competence is periodically checked. Yet even in the United Kingdom, the issue has been a sleeper; and in Canada, Australia and New Zealand, the public seems content with the status quo, although when polled, members of the public support the introduction of some form of regular practice review for doctors (and assume that it already occurs).[6]

Writing in 1988, Jean Robinson, an experienced patient advocate and General Medical Council member, said that '[n]o medical profession in the developed world could have had a body of patients who were more docile and grateful than the British since the formation of the [national] health service'.[7] (One might add Australians and New Zealanders to the roll call of undemanding patients.) Robinson argued that 'the passivity of patients contributed to poor-quality care' and allowed the profession to remain indifferent to tackling competence problems.[8]

Many patient advocates (such as the Canadian group ImPatient for Change) would argue that patients are not passive or unconcerned, but are isolated from each other and face barriers in advocating for change, especially if they are not disease-specific groups supported by pharmaceutical companies.[9] Moreover, patients may think it unlikely that they will personally be affected by a problem doctor, since the odds are less than 1 in 20 that their own doctor will be substandard yet able to continue in practice unchecked. Even if mildly concerned about the current lack of checks of ongoing competence, and frustrated by the general lack of readily accessible information about doctors, the general public may feel powerless to do anything about the situation. Given the track record of delay in implementing change in the UK, even after the highly publicised recommendations of Dame Janet Smith in her Shipman Inquiry report, that sense of powerlessness appears well founded.

Yet there are plenty of examples of the power of motivated health consumers to lobby politicians and secure change. The proposed closure of a local hospital or health service can be a galvanising issue that will lead to petitions and street marches in opposition, and force governments to reconsider the closure.[10] Revelations of injury to multiple patients at the hands of a single doctor or hospital often result in pressure on politicians to establish a public inquiry. Similarly, there have been several instances of lobbying by well-organised consumer groups for public funding of an expensive new medication. In New Zealand, a breast cancer consumer group mounted a successful campaign in the lead-up to the 2008 election, to secure a commitment from the opposition National party to extend funding of the breast cancer medicine Herceptin, which Pharmac (the independent agency charged with evaluating new medicines and recommending whether they should be publicly funded) had recommended only for short-term treatment. The new National Government promptly extended funding upon taking office.[11]

A common feature in the above examples is a tangible cause to rally around: a local hospital, a group of injured patients, or cancer patients deprived of a new medicine. If that cause is fronted by affected patients or their families, putting a human face on the story, it will often gain momentum and support from interest groups with their own barrow to push (such as pharmaceutical companies or political parties). In contrast, the case for recertification of doctors is intangible. Occasionally, when a Shipman, Patel or Bottrill is the spotlight of a public inquiry, there will be stirrings of public discontent about the issue. When an inquiry eventually reports its findings, there are usually multiple recommendations directed at myriad health system deficiencies. The recertification issue tends to drop off the public agenda, since it excites interest mainly from health policy-makers, regulators and the medical profession.

The public is also not demanding more and better-quality comparative information about doctors, and seems uninterested in using the limited information that is available. This is a perplexing conundrum. There is a wealth of comparative information available on the internet about many consumer products (for example, in the retail and banking sectors), and it is well utilised, but that is not yet true of health care. Martin Marshall notes:

> In many ways, it is remarkable that patients do not make more demands for comparative data about health care. We live in an age when most people have free and easy access to information about many aspects of modern life. 'Consumers' are used to either making choices between, or expressing judgements about, a wide variety of products or services.[12]

In the era of the informed, autonomous patient, there is no clamour for comparative information about doctors or the health centres and hospitals where they work, and individual patients tend not to rely on it when choosing providers. Even in the United States, where some reliable comparative information is available, it is utilised primarily by health plans (insurers) and employers (who insure employees), rather than by consumers shopping for their own health care.[13]

There is a growing number of 'physician profiling' websites that rate doctors in the United States and the United Kingdom, but much of the material is advertising or draws on a tiny sample of patients motivated enough to post a comment. Prospective patients are unlikely to find such information of much assistance. As one commentator notes: '[T]he difficulty of more information is knowing what to trust. While Trip Advisor may reliably suggest the best hotel in Amsterdam it may be harder to place your faith in contributions to mybestappendectomy.com.'[14] In a similar vein, Onora O'Neill writes on the topic of informed consent and trust: 'I need to assess what is offered, but may be unable to judge the information for myself.... [W]e need to find trustworthy information.'[15] Raymond Tallis concurs, saying: '[I]f we withdraw trust from doctors, there is nowhere else to invest it.'[16]

In his 1997 book *Demanding Medical Excellence: Doctors and accountability in the information age*, journalist Michael Millenson heralded a new age in which 'patients are gaining an unprecedented opportunity to evaluate [treatment] decisions by taking advantage of newly available, objective information about past medical performance'.[17] Yet even as

Millenson called for patients' trust to be supplemented by information about a physician's performance (such as rate of surgical complications), he noted that '[i]ntimidated by data, we end up choosing hospitals or physicians because they are nearby or maybe because they were used by a friend'.[18]

The results of a 2011 public survey in the United States highlight an intriguing disconnect. On the one hand, 67 per cent of surveyed adults (and 73% of people under 35) agreed they wanted to be able to find more information about doctors online. Yet 49 per cent said they spent more time researching a gift for a family member or friend than researching their primary care doctor. Respondents indicated that they based their choice of doctor on the convenience of the doctor's office location, as opposed to factors such as patient ratings or malpractice records.[19]

One area where information about a doctor's quality of care might be thought likely to influence patient choices is elective cardiac surgery. Since the early 1990s, New York State has mandated publication of data showing mortality following coronary artery bypass surgery, at hospital and individual surgeon level. The data is risk-adjusted and collated by independent experts. It can be trusted. Surely patients facing cardiac surgery would be interested in such data, and would choose surgeons who score well, and avoid those who score poorly? Yet exhaustive studies of the New York and other mandatory reporting regimes provide only limited support for this hypothesis. It seems that the data is primarily used for quality improvement purposes by surgeons and hospitals themselves, and (to a limited extent) by health plans, but not by the public.

This has not deterred UK and US policy-makers from requiring greater information disclosure. In the United Kingdom, as part of the latest round of National Health Service reforms, it is proposed that the Department of Health publish routine GP performance data, including prescribing data.[20] In the United States, under the Affordable Care Act 2010 (the ObamaCare reforms), the Centers for Medicare & Medicaid

Services has been required, from 1 January 2011, to make public certain types of provider information.[21]

Given the lack of evidence that consumers will rely on such information, even in the United States – the home of consumerism and of health care as a marketable commodity – it is hardly surprising that patients in countries with a strong publicly funded health system, such as Australia and New Zealand, have not consistently lobbied for physician profiling.[22] Patient groups may well be supportive of physician profiling, but their energies have been focused on other more pressing issues, such as the implication of major health system reforms.

In summary, the power of consumer voice has yet to be realised when it comes to the availability and use of good-quality information about individual doctors, and arrangements to ensure they have maintained their practice skills. The patients are not demanding change and complacency rules okay.

Overburdened doctors

If undemanding patients allow the status quo to be maintained, unhappy doctors present a more tangible barrier to change. While many doctors support the notion of more information for patients, and will concede privately that current arrangements for renewal of their licence to practise are light-handed, they groan at the prospect of being subject to new requirements to report data and provide evidence of maintenance of competence. For hard-working professionals, such proposals represent an unwanted additional burden and, for some, an affront to their professionalism.

Read any current medical journal or magazine for doctors, and it's easy to gain the impression that a doctor's lot is not a happy one. Surveys of the medical profession regularly paint a gloomy picture, with 50 per cent of British doctors saying they would choose another profession, if they had their time again.²³ Physician discontent is reported in numerous surveys in the United States. Yet there are also contrary indications: the number of applicants to medical school remains high, and there is limited evidence of more physicians retiring early from medical practice. Evidence of job satisfaction emerges in national surveys in the United States, where 8 out of 10 physicians report being satisfied overall with their careers in medicine.²⁴ In a 2011 survey, over 85 per cent of 5193 Australian doctors (including GPs, other specialists and specialists-in-training) reported being moderately or very satisfied with their jobs.²⁵

Whatever the true extent of dissatisfaction amongst doctors, it is not a new phenomenon and is mirrored by dissatisfaction within other professions.²⁶ However, there is no denying that modern doctors are subject to increasing demands. In the United States, physicians refer to managed care and the malpractice crisis as intolerable burdens. David Mechanic locates physician discontent in increased public and patient expectations, and administrative and regulatory controls, which contribute to increased time pressures and erosion of autonomy.²⁷

The demands of central government and increased bureaucracy are pressure points for doctors in the United Kingdom and New Zealand. A former chairman of the BMA bemoaned '[p]aranoid centralism [that] will turn professionals into bean counters answerable not to their patients but to politicians, auditors, commissioners and managers'.²⁸ Law professor Vivienne Harpwood catalogues the ever-increasing demands on British doctors in her book *Medicine, Malpractice and Misapprehensions*, and rejects the popular view that they are 'over-paid, out of control, and under-regulated'.²⁹ In New Zealand, a former chairman of the NZMA described a profession 'under siege from legislators, from regulators, from commissioners and commissions'.³⁰

Similarly dire statements are made by medical leaders in many countries, although one also finds a minority willing to challenge the prevailing view. In Australia, for example, a leading doctor contends that 'medical professionalism is not under threat' and that the real issue is how doctors respond to new ethical challenges, in particular justice and fairness in allocating scarce health resources. Kerry Breen argues that a strong publicly funded health system is one key factor that 'probably insulates Australian doctors from the influences at work in some other developed countries'.[31]

Yet many Australasian doctors would recognise the grim picture of the modern medic in the United Kingdom, painted by Raymond Tallis in his lament *Hippocratic Oaths: Medicine and its discontents*.[32] Tallis writes of the 'appalling burden of responsibility assumed by doctors' leading to 'contemporary discontents'.[33] His thesis is supported by research showing a high level of burnout within the medical profession,[34] contributed to by chronic work stress. Tallis blames the preoccupation with communication skills and informed consent, the imposition of targets and other bureaucratic demands, the multiple pressures of clinical practice (in which the God-like consultant has become the cog-like consultant), the media's portrayal of a 'scandal-hit' medical profession, and the excessive requirements of transparency and accountability, fuelled by (and fuelling) a lack of trust.

Richard Smith, editor of the *British Medical Journal* through the troubled years of the Bristol and Shipman inquiries, observes many of the same developments. However, Smith sees a silver lining in the clouds. He suggests that doctors' unhappiness may be symptomatic of a shift from a 'bogus contract' between patients and doctors, based on inflated ideas of the power of medicine, to a new contract based on a more realistic assessment of the limitations of doctors and medicine.[35] Smith argues that a reappraisal of the patient–doctor relationship is timely and necessary.

Why do overburdened doctors constitute a roadblock to reform? If doctors already feel ground down and disheartened, and if one of the underlying causes of unhappiness is perceived excessive accountability, they will be highly resistant to regulatory reforms that increase accountability by making renewal of their licence to practise medicine subject to competence checks. These sentiments were well captured in the debate prior to enactment of the Health Practitioners Competence Assurance Act 2003. This statute introduced a new model of regulation for all registered health practitioners in New Zealand, with a consistent accountability framework intended to 'protect the health and safety of members of the public by providing for mechanisms to ensure that health practitioners are competent and fit to practise their professions'.[36] Prominent surgeon Ross Blair spoke for many doctors when he said:

> We as surgeons are in danger of becoming mere indentured labourers – where control is shifted into the hands of those with limited knowledge of surgery. As we progressively see a situation where those outside the profession are regulating the profession we are in danger of creating an environment of defensive medicine. . . . [T]he best safeguard for patient care is the professional contract between doctor and patient.[37]

Indentured labourers? The language is strong, and there is no evidence that doctors have been subject to oppressive external regulation since the enactment of the new law. But Blair's view reflected concerns that resonated with many doctors. The medical profession has also had influential allies in raising such worries. In her widely publicised BBC Reith lectures entitled *A Question of Trust*, philosopher Onora O'Neill made a similar argument:

> The pursuit of ever more perfect accountability provides citizens and consumers, patients and parents with more information, more comparisons, more complaints systems; but it also builds a culture of suspicion, low morale, and may ultimately lead to professional cynicism, and . . . public mistrust.[38]

O'Neill sees excessive accountability as 'distorting the proper aims of professional practice',[39] which, for doctors, are to care for their patients. She argues for 'intelligent accountability', by which '[t]hose who are called to account should give an *account* of what they have done, and of their successes or failures, to others who have sufficient time and experience to assess the evidence and report on it'.[40] As we will see in Part 4, this is not a million miles away from the General Medical Council's proposal that doctors develop a portfolio of evidence from their practice, for submission to a 'Responsible Officer' to evaluate and report to the GMC prior to a revalidation decision.

For busy, overworked doctors, any proposal that involves more paperwork and reporting to external bodies is the last straw. This has been a theme of medical professional resistance to the GMC's revalidation proposals in the aftermath of the Shipman Inquiry. It was also evident in New Zealand in 2006, when a fairly modest pilot by the Medical Council, to test the proposed introduction of mandatory 360-degree feedback from a sample of a doctor's patients and colleagues, was criticised as unduly onerous and – in a common refrain whenever multisource feedback is mooted – statistically flawed.

Nor is it simply a matter of excessive burdens. For some doctors, it is demotivating to be told that they must prove their ongoing competence, since it suggests a lack of trust in their own professionalism. Trust is a complex motivator for professionals. In the debate surrounding the introduction of the new 'Quality Outcomes Framework' for general practice in the United Kingdom, one of the telling points made by critics was that the contractually rewarded activities ('payment for results') might undermine self-motivation to provide high-quality care for patients.[41] Doctors will respond to price signals, and will also no doubt jump through whatever regulatory hoops are required of them. But targets and incentives can carry a hidden cost: 'In the end carrots and sticks may make general practitioners behave more like donkeys than doctors.'[42] If that happens, as a society we may end up paying a high price.

Of course, one can respond that increasing accountability is a worldwide phenomenon that affects all professionals, not just doctors.[43]

However, the above considerations suggest reasons why doctors may resist requirements to report more data and undergo competence checks. They are well placed to oppose reforms. There is a global shortage of doctors. In developed countries, there is a rising tide of patients presenting with complex medical problems. Fiscally constrained Health Ministers are trying to free doctors from red tape and paperwork so they can focus on delivering care to such patients. Against this backdrop, overburdened doctors (and their politically savvy representatives) are able to call in political capital. They represent a major roadblock to change.

Reluctant regulators

Most patients lack the time, energy or commitment to seek out information about doctors and lobby for more effective checks on their competence. Doctors themselves are unlikely to push for rigorous recertification processes. Yet medical boards are charged by Parliament with the task of ensuring that doctors remain competent and fit to practise. How effective are they at doing so?

In my observation, boards do a good job in setting and enforcing high ethical standards for medical practitioners, in areas such as appropriate boundaries with patients, and doctors in commerce; are generally adept at supporting and monitoring doctors with health problems to return to safe practice, if possible; but struggle with cases where an employer or colleague raises concerns of poor performance. The historical failure of the General Medical Council to tackle professional performance is well documented. Lay member Margaret Stacey, who served on the GMC from 1976 to 1984, wrote that the Council 'has never really ensured the continuing competence of registered practitioners' and 'on balance resolved the many tensions it faced in regulating the profession in favour of the profession rather than the public'.[44] It is a criticism that can be levelled at many professional regulators.

Medical boards inevitably walk a fine line between guiding and policing good medical practice. The contrasting approaches are nicely illustrated by comparing the stated mission of the College of Physicians & Surgeons of Alberta – 'Serving the public by guiding the medical profession' – with the declared purpose of the United Kingdom General Medical Council – 'to protect, promote and maintain the health and safety of the public by ensuring proper standards in the practice of medicine'.

Boards have to balance public and professional concerns. The balancing act is well described by Carl Ameringer in his definitive United States study *State Medical Boards and the Politics of Public Protection*.[45] Given their composition of predominantly medical members, boards have tended to err on the side of remediation and rehabilitation of physicians rather than formal discipline and public disclosure. Ameringer argues that, in relation to incompetent practitioners, boards embraced quality improvement ideas and became 'guide dogs', not 'watchdogs'. In a case study of Maryland, he writes: 'Because the focus of peer review was education rather than punishment, reviewers failed to weed out incompetent practitioners, as did the state board whose members, all physicians, favored rehabilitation.'[46]

The theme is a familiar one, not lost on me as the former head of a co-regulatory agency[47] charged with protecting patients' rights, where we adopted the motto 'Learning, not lynching, Resolution, not retribution'. Regulators in the health arena face all sorts of subtle pressures to take a lenient approach, particularly when the community is short of health practitioners. Isn't a mediocre doctor who promises to do better next time better than no doctor at all? Rehabilitation is a worthy goal, but when it is pursued at the expense of public protection and accountability, the price may be too high.

These tensions are evident in the history of medical boards in the United Kingdom, Canada, Australia and New Zealand. In the Antipodean jurisdictions, responsibility for formal discipline has been removed from health practitioner boards, but there remains a clear public protective mandate in relation to registration and oversight of health practitioners. The first objective of Australia's new health practitioner national registration and accreditation scheme is 'to provide for the protection of the public by ensuring that only health practitioners who are suitably trained and qualified to practise in a competent and ethical manner are registered'. However, the statute makes it clear that the public protective goal is to be juggled with other statutory objectives, which relate to facilitation of workforce mobility, education and training, and access to services.[48]

Public safety was a key factor in Australia's law reform. Media statements from the Council of Australian Governments emphasised that the new arrangements would provide greater safeguards for the public. Concerns about lax regulatory practice had emerged during the Queensland Inquiry into surgeon Patel. The Commission of Inquiry stated that a medical board is not excused from performing its statutory role because it lacks resources.[49] The Commission also noted that concern for the rights of the doctor does not justify a board allowing a real risk to patients to continue until a thorough investigation has taken place or until evidence is tested in a contested hearing.[50]

Medical boards are often small bureaucracies with heavy workloads and competing demands. Inevitably, they are vulnerable to criticism for being slow and reactive, features that were evident in two major inquiries I undertook in New Zealand where the Medical Council had been alerted to concerns about poorly performing practitioners. Long delays were a feature of the Council's competence review of the problem surgeon in the Tauranga Hospitals Inquiry;[51] unsatisfactory registration practices and poor information-sharing between Australian state medical boards and the Council were evident in the case of Dr Roman Hasil, the Slovakian gynaecologist who had practised in Australia before he came to Wanganui Hospital and performed tubal ligations with a high failure rate of 25 per cent.[52]

The New South Wales and New Zealand boards have developed performance assessment processes to remediate practitioners about whom performance concerns have been flagged. These constructive processes have contributed to a decline in disciplinary proceedings and helped rehabilitate some doctors.[53] However, the processes are shrouded in secrecy and, despite the confidential and remedial approach, are often bitterly contested by doctors. In my experience, when performance concerns are raised about an individual doctor, boards are sometimes backed into a corner by medical defence counsel. Boards seem reluctant to exercise powers to suspend or restrict a doctor's practice, and to ensure that the public register accurately reflects any restrictions. Cases are often sent down a health or performance assessment track, with a focus on rehabilitation of the doctor, arguably without proper regard to the need for public protection and accountability to affected patients.

An independent review of the Medical Council of New Zealand in 2010 endorsed its rehabilitative approach, but warned of the risk that 'cases that should be considered under the conduct procedures are dealt with as competence cases' and of 'too comfortable a relationship developing between the profession and the regulator'.[54] The review also noted the need for greater transparency to ensure 'accountability and maintaining public confidence in the system of regulation of doctors in New Zealand' and cautioned against adoption of priorities that 'appear to be based on government [workforce] priorities rather than strict public protection'.[55]

Medical boards are often decidedly risk-averse, by which I mean an aversion to organisational risk (such as the threat of judicial review of board action by defence lawyers) rather than an aversion to patient risk. The voice of the doctor, amplified by legal representation, is usually louder and more articulate than the voice of the patient, and it often seems that backing away from strong measures is the 'safer' approach. Furthermore, harm to the practitioner, in the form of suspension, is immediate and quantifiable, while risk of harm to the public is distant and uncertain.

Members who have served on medical boards testify to regulatory conservatism and inertia, and the need to placate medical members with strong allegiances to their profession. (Unsurprisingly, those who give accounts of efforts to coax colleagues to take a firmer line – for example, in responding to poorly performing doctors – tend to show themselves in a favourable light.) A fascinating history of the General Medical Council in turbulent times in the 1980s and 1990s, by former President Donald Irvine, recounts the public and political pressures that finally forced the GMC to undergo reform and tackle competence issues.[56]

Even the reformed General Medical Council, which has probably faced more intense media and public scrutiny than any other medical regulator in the western world, is struggling to be a rigorous regulator. It continues to face fierce criticism in the media. Dame Janet Smith has expressed 'despair about the GMC ever getting it right', citing 'a reluctance to be tough' and strike off problem doctors.[57] On a BBC Radio 4 documentary in early 2011, Peter Walsh, the Chief Executive of the lobby group AvMA, Action against Medical Accidents, said: 'We don't get the really robust and consistent regulation of doctors that we all want to see. . . . We believe that in the vast majority of cases, they get things right. But in a handful of serious cases with huge public interest implications, they get it very badly wrong.'[58] On the same programme, doctors from Doctors4Justice were quoted describing the GMC as 'a law unto themselves'. This sort of criticism from both sides will be familiar to anyone who has worked in the world of medical regulation or patient complaints.

To return to my opening question: how effective are medical boards at ensuring that doctors remain competent and fit to practise? In my assessment, they do a passable job of reacting to concerns about poor performance, but have yet to demonstrate rigour in proactively checking doctors' competence. They are 'reluctant regulators' whose passive resistance to change has slowed progress towards the goal of assuredly good doctors expected by the public.

Medical culture

The greatest roadblock to change is not the patients, the doctors, or the medical regulators, but the culture of medicine, which influences the behaviour of all those players. Culture, sometimes defined as 'the way we do things around here', has become ubiquitous in any discussion of the health system. Read the burgeoning patient safety and healthcare quality improvement literature, and you will find reference time and again to the importance of cultural change, and how failure to take account of the complex patterns of behaviour in the health system will doom any imposed initiative to failure. The same is true of regulatory initiatives that pay insufficient heed to medical culture, such as the introduction in 2003 of an 80 work hours per week maximum for junior doctors or 'residents' in US hospitals.[59] In the words of the slogan, 'Culture eats strategy for breakfast every time'.

Medical culture is probably the most powerful influence on the way that doctors practise.[60] It has contributed in many positive ways to the remarkable march of progress of modern medicine. Tallis, in a powerful critique of the 'enemies of progress', criticises '[t]he collective amnesia of how things were in the past – and an upward calibration of expectation and a downwards regulation of tolerance to imperfections'.[61] The medical miracles we now take for granted are born of a remarkable culture of scientific inquiry, emphasis on teaching and learning, teamwork, audit and peer review, and commitment to patient care. Irvine, sometimes a fierce critic of his own profession, writes that '[o]verwhelmingly the medical culture has been, and still is, founded on the fact that the majority of doctors want to do their best for their patients ... frequently at the expense of a doctor's own interests and personal needs'.[62]

However, culture can also inhibit progress. As noted by Jean Robinson: 'The culture [of medicine] has also decreed that once a doctor has been trained, he or she is competent unless proved otherwise, and that the clinician will naturally update knowledge and skills as required by a process of osmosis, without extra formal training or reaccreditation being required.'[63] Professionalism, the 'internal morality' of medicine,[64] and self-regulation are seen as the best safeguards of patients and of the competence of doctors. Professional colleges *have* responded to the need to develop maintenance of professional standards (MOPS) programmes. But there is strong resistance to rules imposed from outside the profession, so-called 'external regulation', which is regarded as unnecessary, excessive and counterproductive.

In everyday clinical practice, deeply embedded culture sometimes frustrates the attainment of worthy professional goals. Culture takes a long time to change, and doctors remain highly resistant to being judged by anyone other than their own peers, through peer review and audit processes. They question why more regulation is needed. One can understand doctors' distrust of legislative reforms. New Zealand and the United Kingdom have both been intense laboratories for reform of the publicly funded health system over the past 20 years. The reforms have been labour-intensive for doctors and have yielded decidedly mixed results for the public. The medical profession has been highly critical of the politicians and policy-makers who have implemented change without proper testing and evaluation. Similarly, when micro reforms are proposed, doctors are wary of unproven strategies such as publication of comparative quality information or enhanced checks on doctors' performance.

Something deeper is going on here than aversion to accountability or a fear of being found wanting. Many doctors bring to this debate the cautious scepticism of the scientist combined with the deep-seated emotions of the practitioner of the art of medicine. Loyalty to one's peers runs very deep in the medical profession, at least when there is a perceived external threat. The concept of a loyal 'brotherhood' is captured in the venerated Hippocratic Oath, which contains the pledge (albeit to one's teachers, rather than one's colleagues): 'To hold him who has taught me this art as equal to my parents and to live my life in partnership with him . . .'[65]

How does loyalty show itself? Although doctors generally set high standards in their clinical practice, and aim for perfection, they are well aware of their own fallibility. Most doctors will make a serious mistake during their medical career that exposes a patient to the risk of harm, and many will recall the experience as a private nightmare, especially if their patient suffered harm. So, on learning of another doctor's mistake, their instinctive reaction is likely to be the thought: 'There but for the grace of God, go I.' Doctors have a strong sense of empathy for the fellow practitioner who makes a mistake.

The imaginative feat of standing in another doctor's shoes, understanding how an error may have occurred, and empathising with their plight, has much to commend it.[66] Less commendable is the tendency for empathy, or a misplaced sense of loyalty, to lead to a loss of objectivity. This can cloud doctors' judgement about the implications of their colleague's error, both for the affected patient and for future patients. It is often easier to do nothing, perhaps justifying inaction on the basis that it was a one-off error by an otherwise competent doctor. That stance may be understandable if it follows the observation of a colleague's mistake on a single occasion. But it is an inexcusable response when poor practice is observed on several occasions.

Some doctors do take action, by approaching the colleague directly, or reporting concerns to the doctor's employer, clinical director, or work partner. Sometimes this will lead to an effective resolution, but frequently the intervenor will be rebuffed or receive a perfunctory response. The doctor at issue may deny there is a problem and respond defensively or threaten to bring in a lawyer. Unless the employer is willing to pursue the matter, a stalemate may result. If the problem behaviour endures, the intervenor will face a dilemma: whether to report to an external authority. Whistle-blowers who air their concerns outside their organisation risk professional ostracism.[67] It may be tempting to place an unresolved problem in the too-hard basket, rather than make an external report, for fear of being seen to 'dob in' another doctor.

I recall the case of a surgeon whose substandard care caused serious harm to several patients, resulting in complaints, investigations, disciplinary findings of professional misconduct, mandatory retraining, and the shame of being publicly named. A thoughtful leader of the surgical profession in New Zealand, bemoaning the surgeon's plight, said to me as an aside, 'Of course, we all knew that he wasn't really up to scratch.'[68] I was dumbfounded. The failure of surgical colleagues to act was a disservice to the surgeon and, most importantly, his patients. It deprived a surgeon of the opportunity to remedy his deficiencies and protect his reputation before it was too late, and it placed his patients at risk.

It is remarkable that these attitudes endure in the twenty-first century. One would expect the 'club culture' identified by Ian Kennedy during the Bristol Inquiry[69] to be far less dominant, given the heterogeneity of the modern medical profession. One need only look at a class of medical students in New Zealand to see that they are no longer a homogeneous collection of white males, often the scions of medical families and graduates from a select group of private schools. Instead, at least half the students are female, and classes now have much more diverse ethnic origins. Nor is this a recent phenomenon – I have lectured to classes at Auckland and Otago medical schools for over a decade and observed a similar pattern. The medical student body has changed and is much more representative of the general population.[70] They feed into a New Zealand medical workforce that is changing significantly owing to the high proportion of overseas-trained doctors.[71] Similar patterns are occurring in Australia, Canada and the United Kingdom.

Yet the remnants of a club culture linger on. Old habits and attitudes die hard. Doctors join a medical tribe that has tough initiation rites.[72] The process of socialisation begins at medical school and continues during their training as junior doctors in hospital.[73] They develop a 'professional protective carapace'.[74] Students and trainees learn to keep their heads down and to know their place within the medical hierarchy. They are sometimes troubled by witnessing inappropriate behaviour by senior doctors towards patients, but may feel powerless to challenge it and ashamed by their reluctance to intervene.[75]

Despite the much greater emphasis on medical ethics and patients' rights nowadays, inappropriate behaviour may still go unchallenged or unreported. That is particularly so when concerns relate to skills and competence – the inevitable shades of grey mean that questionable performance often goes unquestioned, putting patients at risk. Norms of professional etiquette, buttressed by uncertainty and recognition of shared fallibility and vulnerability, lead to a reticence to judge.[76]

Over a quarter of a century ago, McIntyre and Popper called for a new ethos in medicine, in which error is admitted and learnt from, not covered up and denied.[77] They argued that the profession's effective monopoly over the right to practise carries with it a duty to judge the error of colleagues. Yet their vision of rigorous self-regulation remains largely aspirational.

In a decade of investigating patient complaints, including a minority involving poorly performing medical practitioners, I saw a continued reluctance on the part of doctors to judge the errors of colleagues. I was mystified by what I considered an irrational response, given the strong emphasis in the patient complaints system on learning rather than punishment. My thesis, extolled *ad nauseam* to medical audiences, was that the relatively modest consequences of my 'opinions' as Health and Disability Commissioner (with individual providers not being publicly named or shamed, and formal discipline occurring rarely)[78] meant that doctors should be willing to criticise and take action in the face of poor performance.

But I underestimated the cultural factors of loyalty and empathy, and the point that criticism from an external inquiry body leads to feelings of shame in the subject practitioner.[79] Furthermore, those doctors who were willing to provide expert advice to an external inquiry became the target of potential criticism by raising their heads above the parapet. I saw this most vividly in an investigation of the care of a 50-year-old patient during a 40-hour admission that ended in his death at Wellington

Hospital in 2004. On the basis of independent advice from named expert physicians, my highly publicised report identified serious failings in the care provided by unnamed doctors and nurses, and the named hospital.[80]

The medical advisors were fiercely criticised by the President of the New Zealand Medical Association, in a speech revealingly entitled 'Loyal to the Profession of Medicine and Just and Generous to its Members'.[81] He accused them of 'enthusiastic, but potentially arrogant . . . expertise or ignorance' and called on the profession to 'alert others to the path of arrogance of ignorance'. I have rebutted this criticism elsewhere.[82] My concern here is that the denigration of experts reinforces a 'closed shop' culture within medicine. I saw first-hand that it made medical experts reluctant to advise an inquiry on standards of care.[83] Why rock the boat by criticising one's peers (who are almost invariably not identified in the published investigation report, unlike the expert advisors) and risk public censure oneself?

Statutory decision-makers in health care, as in other fields, must expect to have their reasons for decision critiqued. Independent scrutiny of an expert's published advice is an important safeguard. But there is no excuse for the denigration of experts.[84] As Charlotte Paul and Linda Holloway, who served as medical advisors to the Cartwright Inquiry, wrote in the aftermath of that inquiry: 'Is anyone involved in a critical assessment of a colleague's work to be regarded as a proper target for . . . denigration? Only by withstanding such attacks and refusing to become cynical can we assist society in finding better ways to deal with error in medicine.'[85]

In less formal situations, doctors are much freer with their criticism. A curious paradox is evident. I saw numerous cases where a doctor, consulted for a second opinion by a patient concerned about the standard of medical care provided by an earlier doctor, would volubly criticise the former doctor's standards, often without the benefit of the full facts. Naturally, these sorts of casual comments sometimes precipitated a patient's complaint. Yet when it came to confronting the former doctor directly, reporting concerns to an employer or the Medical Council, or giving evidence to an inquiry body, doctors seemed much less sure of their ground. In the next section, I discuss some of the ways in which the law unwittingly reinforces a self-protective medical culture.

Why do members of a profession dedicated to caring for patients find it so difficult to respond adequately to competence concerns? If the possession and maintenance of special skills is the hallmark of a medical professional, why is poor performance so often tolerated until complaints, or serious harm to a patient, forces someone to act? Why is a subject that could (and, in my view, should) be called 'protect-a-patient' instead reframed as 'dob-a-doc'? Why is it 'not done' for a doctor to report suspicions about a colleague to the authorities, as Dame Janet Smith noted in the Shipman Inquiry?[86] Why does one still hear the following sort of comment, made by a senior doctor in a modern English teaching hospital?

> There's definitely a culture against doing this kind of thing. There's a definite culture where you shouldn't implicate other doctors when things go wrong because it's not in their interests, despite being in the interests of safety and improvement.[87]

I do not accept the view that there is 'a culture of cover-up' in medicine.[88] I think that is a simplistic view that implies conspiracy on the part of doctors and the medical profession. The way in which doctors act when confronted with apparent error is complex. Doctors enact specific rituals, particularly in hospital settings. A mortality and morbidity (M & M) meeting, at which a senior doctor describes a recent case and invites comments from colleagues, is an important mechanism for learning from mistakes. Charles Bosk, observing the surgical service in a major American teaching hospital in the 1970s, noted that even this 'public confessional' actually maintained 'a conspiracy of silence', since individuals involved in the case were not identified and professional responsibility was treated as an individual but not a corporate responsibility.[89] Atul Gawande describes contemporary US surgical M & M meetings in similar terms: '[S]urgeons maintain an old-fashioned sense of hierarchy. When things go wrong, the attending [the staff surgeon in charge of the case] is expected to take full responsibility.'[90] In New Zealand and Australia, at least for medical M & M meetings, the format is less hierarchical and the focus is on systems problems and how to solve them.[91]

In ground-breaking research in 1990, American sociologist Marilynn Rosenthal interviewed 60 doctors, nurses, managers and officials in the United Kingdom, and 40 in Sweden. Rosenthal published her findings in her book *The Incompetent Doctor: Behind closed doors*.[92] Key themes emerged at interview. Doctors approach the issue of mistakes and mishaps with an acute consciousness of the permanent uncertainty of medical work, and recognise that 'necessary fallibility' is an intrinsic part of the practice of medicine. Their reluctance to judge colleagues stems from a sense of shared personal vulnerability and an impulse to understand and forgive, especially if the colleague expresses remorse. This is compounded by a tacit norm of non-criticism, together with a commonly held view that only the profession can judge the clinical behaviour of its members.[93]

Rosenthal identified a repertoire of informal mechanisms used to try to sort out problems in a low-key way. They include the 'terribly quiet chat', when a close senior colleague confides that there are concerns and seeks to persuade the doctor to change their problem behaviour. Other informal means include 'workaround' or diverting patient flow from the problem doctor; providing protective support to help the doctor continue to work; 'exporting the problem'; and 'the dignity bribe' of early retirement and financial compensation.

These are familiar techniques to anyone who has undertaken inquiries into patient harm caused by problem doctors. At Bundaberg Hospital in 2005, intensivists and nurses resorted to hiding patients from Dr Patel, in an extreme example of workaround.[94] As occurred in that case, diversion may be a desperate measure taken when colleagues see that management is unwilling or unable to deal with a problem effectively. Sometimes the quiet chat or corridor conversation may be a crucial intervention that persuades a problem doctor to seek help, limit their practice, or take remedial steps. But Rosenthal's interviewees noted that it was often an ineffective response, leading to a stalemate, with the problem doctor being marginalised but continuing to work.

Clearly, it is a very difficult thing to tackle a medical colleague about poor performance, let alone to make a report to an employing manager, college, or medical board. The problem of the poorly performing colleague arises in many workplaces. Think of the university lecturer who is known to rehash outdated lectures and to be panned by students every year. Frequently the response from senior colleagues or management is to have a gentle chat to the problem lecturer, but seldom is any decisive remedial action taken. Such misplaced collegial loyalty is not confined to the medical profession. However, the stakes are higher in health care than in most other work environments. The problem doctor may cause serious harm to patients.

In the past, it was considered a breach of professional etiquette for one doctor to disparage the work of another doctor; in the United Kingdom, the professional 'Blue Book' forbade such conduct.[95] But in recent decades, the attitude of regulators has changed, and professional guidelines spell out that doctors have an ethical duty to inform an appropriate person or body about a colleague whose performance appears to be deficient. Evidence is emerging in the United Kingdom of a greater willingness amongst doctors to report concerns.[96]

The New Zealand Medical Council is refreshingly clear in its 2010 Statement *What to do when you have concerns about a colleague*.[97] The Statement begins by saying: 'Doctors have an ethical responsibility to protect patients from risk of harm posed by a colleague's conduct, performance or health. Patient safety should come first at all times.'

The Council acknowledges how difficult it is to raise concerns about a colleague, noting: 'You may be reluctant to act on concerns for a variety of reasons, for example because you fear that it may cause problems for colleagues, adversely affect working relationships, have a negative impact on your career or result in a complaint about you.' Interestingly, the Statement hints that failure to report concerns about a colleague may itself lead the non-reporter to have the omission considered by medical authorities; but reporting a colleague is not mandatory, at least in relation to competence, as opposed to health, concerns.[98]

Statements such as these reflect an effort by regulators to coax doctors to take action when they have concerns about substandard practice by a colleague. In my view, placing the emphasis on a doctor's ethical responsibility is more likely to encourage reporting than external regulation. Interestingly, the New Zealand Code gives patients the right to compliance, by health practitioners, with 'legal, professional, *ethical*, and other relevant standards'.[99] The Code thus affirms the setting of ethical standards by health professions, but gives patients a means of redress (by making a complaint) if practitioners fail to comply.

However, other countries have gone further. In Australia, in response to concerns following the cases of surgeon Jayant Patel in Queensland and gynaecologist Graeme Reeves in New South Wales, all states and territories have enacted the Health Practitioner Regulation National Law 2009, which includes a mandatory duty to report competence concerns. A registered health practitioner who, in the course of practising his or her profession, forms a reasonable belief that another health practitioner has behaved in a way that constitutes 'notifiable conduct' must promptly notify the national regulator. Notifiable conduct includes practice while intoxicated by alcohol or drugs, and sexual misconduct; placing the public 'at risk of substantial harm ... because the practitioner has an impairment'; and placing the public 'at risk of harm because the practitioner has practised the profession in a way that constitutes a significant departure from accepted professional standards'.[100]

I am sceptical about whether mandatory reporting will alter the entrenched behaviour of health practitioners. It smacks of politicians seeking to 'do something' in response to a medical scandal. Although it sends an important signal of the importance that the public places on health practitioners taking decisive action in the face of seriously incompetent practice by a colleague, it risks encouraging doctors to conceal impairments rather than seek help. There will inevitably be debate as to when the threshold of a 'significant departure from accepted professional standards' has been reached and what is a 'reasonable belief'.[101] The law is a blunt tool to change medical culture, which represents a formidable barrier to change.

Legal constraints

The law is not an actor in this medical drama, in the way that undemanding patients, overburdened doctors and reluctant regulators are. Nor is it as all-pervasive an influence as medical culture. Yet the law undeniably restrains effective action on the problem of problem doctors. Roadblock may be putting it too strongly, but there are several ways in which the law and legal constraints impede solutions in this area.

The 'Bolam' rule and expert advice

First, by clinging to the traditional *Bolam* test, the law allows a wide margin of deference in determining what is 'reasonable' practice. Under the *Bolam* standard, which still largely holds sway in Australia, New Zealand and the United Kingdom, the adequacy of medical practice is determined on the basis of professional opinion, rather than patient expectations.[102] 'Reasonable' practice means acting in accordance with what a 'responsible body' of medical opinion would consider acceptable practice in the circumstances. Even if the majority of peers would set a higher standard, it is sufficient to meet the minimum regarded as acceptable by a minority. Thus, according to *Bolam*, if most doctors would prescribe prophylactic antibiotics, but not doing so is regarded as acceptable practice, a doctor's non-prescription will not amount to negligence.

Judges have nibbled away at the edges of the *Bolam* rule, insisting that it is ultimately for the courts, rather than the profession itself, to determine whether a reasonable standard of care has been achieved. In the *Bolitho* case, the House of Lords noted that, even in the face of unanimous clinical opinion that a certain practice is reasonable, if there is a logical flaw in that practice (for example, if a simple precaution, such as a physical examination or a diagnostic test, could avert harm to the patient), the court may form its own view and find a practitioner negligent.[103]

In Australia, legislation has codified the *Bolam* rule (subject to the *Bolitho* exception), to allay doctors' fears of indeterminate liability for negligence.[104] No such step has been taken in New Zealand, where accident compensation cover for 'treatment injury' substitutes for common law claims for medical negligence. The standard of care does, however, frequently arise in Health and Disability Commissioner investigations of whether a provider met the Code duty to provide services 'with reasonable care and skill'.[105] There is no automatic application of the *Bolam* rule. Expert advice is highly persuasive, at least in relation to questions of assessment, diagnosis and treatment, but the Commissioner will scrutinise the evidence to see whether accepted practice reflects custom rather than care, in which case a breach of standards may be found.[106] For example, even if it is accepted practice for a GP to leave a patient with chest pains to arrange his own transport from a general practice to a hospital emergency department, the GP's failure to arrange an ambulance may result in a finding of failure to exercise reasonable care.[107]

Expert evidence presents a range of problems. There is often a low level of agreement between physicians asked to review quality of care,[108] reflecting the subjective assessments of experts on the normative issue of the appropriate standard of care in the circumstances. This may come as a surprise to members of the public, who imagine that objective standards can be applied to determine whether a doctor provided appropriate care. The quality of advice from experts can also be highly variable.[109] Skilful defence counsel need only find an expert willing to say that a doctor's acts or omission were reasonable, in order to sow seeds of doubt about what might at first blush appear negligent practice. There tends to be no shortage of experts for the defence, no doubt reflecting the cultural factors of uncertainty, fallibility and empathy.

As noted earlier, experts who are willing to criticise a doctor's practice are likely to be challenged and have their own credentials criticised.[110] In my experience, expert medical witnesses hesitate to criticise a peer's conduct as below par unless it is clearly egregious. They may be concerned about the personal repercussions of doing so. Where criticism is expressed, it is often so mild (for example, describing the care as 'suboptimal') that the subject doctor can still claim to have met the *Bolam* standard of 'reasonable' practice. If the criticism is more strongly worded, the expert is frequently said to be applying a 'gold standard', or the argument is made that a single failure is not generalisable.

An expert advisor may self-censure to avoid any legal back and forth, leading to a report that understates any deficiencies. Experts who have initially been critical may feel pressured to modify their criticism as a result of submissions by adversely affected parties. If modification of initial criticism leads to a more informed and balanced report, so much the better. However, one would not expect the movement to be all one way. Yet in my experience of HDC investigations, it is far more common for criticism to be muted as a result of the submissions made by a health practitioner in response to a provisional (adverse) opinion, than for criticism to be bolstered following submissions from an aggrieved patient or complainant. Research on a small sample of reported HDC decisions confirms that impression.[111] It probably reflects both reticence to judge and the reality that practitioners are funded by insurers to obtain advice to challenge a provisional opinion, whereas complainants have to pay out of pocket for such advice.

The upshot is that, even in cases that seem clear-cut, where medical experts have initially criticised care as substandard, what is 'reasonable' practice takes on shades of grey.

Hindsight and outcome bias

Other factors also come into play. Since reviews are necessarily retrospective, there is always a risk of hindsight bias (looking through 'the retrospectoscope') and outcome bias (the reviewers' knowledge of the patient's adverse outcome), and any criticism may be discounted on this basis.[112] The possibility of hindsight and outcome bias needs to be acknowledged and guarded against (for example, by attempting to blind the reviewer to the outcome). These are important concerns that highlight the need for care in inquiring into the quality of health care, but they do not mean that regulators and external inquiry bodies should 'butt out' and leave the review task to in-house mortality and morbidity meetings.

There is a fundamental difference between medicine and law.[113] Medicine is essentially concerned with the prognosis for the patient – looking at treatment options having established a diagnosis. Law, in particular a legal inquiry, is necessarily retrospective. It is impossible to hold an inquiry in advance. Of necessity, the inquirer looks back at events that have already occurred and asks what health care the patient *should* have received. That is a normative, rather than a moralistic, question. (It includes consideration of the steps a doctor should have taken prospectively, to minimise the known risks of a serious outcome.) Furthermore, when a bad outcome does eventuate, and the patient dies or suffers major harm, it is all the more important to learn whether other patients may be at risk of harm from substandard practice.

Natural justice

A second confounding legal factor is the impact of the requirements of natural justice and fairness on an inquiry process. It is all too easy for reviewers to leap to adverse conclusions, particularly when a patient has died or suffered terrible harm. Decision-makers may misstate basic facts, leading to unsound conclusions. Natural justice (including the requirement of *audi alteram partem*, to hear the other side) helps guard against unwarranted criticism by requiring that any proposed adverse comment be released to affected persons, giving them an opportunity to respond.[114] The courts have noted that independent examination of the conduct of a medical practitioner is 'exactly the sort of situation in which high standards of procedural fairness are expected, to support the process of making the careful professional judgments that are called for'.[115]

Even when a trail of harm to patients is clearly established, there will usually be some colleagues who leap to the defence of the doctor whose performance is under fire. When the appalling track record of Dr Patel at Bundaberg Hospital was finally exposed publicly, a manager of the hospital wrote to the local newspaper decrying the lack of natural justice for the individual surgeon: 'Dr Patel is an industrious surgeon who has spent many years working to improve the lives of ordinary people in both the United States and Australia. He deserves a fair go.'[116]

Doctors whose employment and reputation are potentially in jeopardy certainly deserve 'a fair go'. The requirement to act fairly is an important consideration for any hospital that employs or gives 'visiting privileges' to a doctor. But excessive consultation and legal process may impede establishing whether there truly is a performance problem and, if so, taking the necessary steps to remedy it.

As an example, the contractual provisions in the multi-employer collective agreement for senior doctors in New Zealand public hospitals prescribe exhaustive requirements relating to investigations of clinical practice.[117] The affected employed doctor is to be told the identity of the person raising the performance concern, and to be consulted about whether an investigation proceeds and, if so, its terms of reference. Employers may impose only the 'absolute minimum' restrictions on the doctor's clinical practice in order to avoid patient harm; the restrictions lapse after three weeks unless a panel of three senior practitioners (at least one nominated by the doctor) agrees otherwise, and lapse after three months unless a second panel of three senior practitioners (at least two nominated by the doctor) endorses the need for continued restrictions. It is not hard to imagine that colleagues might be deterred from reporting concerns, if their identity is to be revealed, and employers might wilt in the face of such rigmarole.

Hospitals are supposed to have good clinical governance systems in place, including incident reporting systems, clinical audit, and credentialling of doctors. Inevitably, questions about clinical performance will occasionally come to light. Such cases are best resolved by prompt, robust internal investigations. To quote one of my own decisions: 'The interests of patients and clinicians will be better served if issues relating to competence are dealt with firmly and fairly in the workplace, before they escalate, patients (and the clinician's reputation) are harmed, and external agencies become involved.'[118]

Where an internal investigation establishes that a doctor is not performing at the expected standard, an employer may need to limit their scope of practice, until the underlying competence or communication issues can be remedied. If remediation is not possible, the employer may have to take the ultimate step of dismissal or withdrawal of visiting privileges. Any of these steps may lead to legal challenges from the affected doctor, especially when employment contracts carefully circumscribe the employer's actions. It is obviously appropriate that employment tribunals and courts are zealous in protecting the rights of practitioners whose livelihood is at risk. Courts invariably speak of the need for high standards of procedural fairness in such situations.[119] But the law struggles to find a balance between the rights of individual practitioners and patient safety.

I recall my Tauranga Hospitals Inquiry, which considered whether two private hospitals and a public hospital took adequate steps to ensure that surgeon Ian Breeze was competent to practise surgery and to respond to concerns about his work (including his rate of postoperative complications). Only one hospital had acted swiftly to restrict his clinical practice. I commented: 'Hospitals must have in place a clear mechanism for dealing decisively with concerns about an employee's competence. Although employees are entitled to be treated fairly, hospitals cannot allow patient safety to be jeopardized while employees and their lawyers squabble about legal rights.'[120]

Other decision-makers have made the same point. In an employment case in the airline industry, Judge Finnigan noted: '[W]here safety is genuinely involved in the operations of an employer, it is not just another ingredient in the mix, another factor to be taken into account. Safety issues have a status of their own.'[121] What is true of air travel – with which parallels are often drawn by healthcare quality experts – is equally true of patient safety in hospitals.

Comments such as these might be expected to embolden hospital boards to err on the side of patient safety in tackling performance problems amongst clinical staff. However, boards are wary of being found liable in damages for wrongful dismissal and the adverse publicity attendant on such findings. New Zealand district health board chief executives have admitted to being risk-averse in such situations, having watched other boards be caned by the courts for acting too hastily in dismissing a problem doctor.[122] One private hospital board chairman told the media: 'If we wrongfully withdrew access, we would have to ask whether they could take legal action against us. We could be sued for ruining a career.'[123]

Legal advisors for hospitals and health boards are likely to counsel employers to take a cautious approach, which often means that a doctor is 'counselled' and 'monitored', but the underlying problems fester. As a result, employers are quite often timorous. A common strategy is to export the problem. As I noted in my Whanganui District Health Board Inquiry: 'The tendency in many organisations is to use informal mechanisms to deal with problems of poor performance or failure, such as finding a way for a "problem doctor" to exit quietly without any formal action. The result is that problems get moved around the health system rather than being tackled and resolved.'[124]

Scope of review

A separate legal issue is the scope of any review of a doctor's practice, and the admissibility of evidence of past problems. It is obviously not a straightforward matter to establish that substandard care was provided on a single occasion. Allegations of medical negligence are difficult to sustain, even where there has been questionable practice.[125] But it is even more difficult to prove a pattern of substandard practice establishing incompetence or poor performance by a doctor. Requirements of fairness to the individual practitioner whose work is under scrutiny mean that each case is looked at in isolation.

This blinkered legal approach makes it very difficult for a court, complaint commission, disciplinary tribunal or inquiry body to see the overall picture of a doctor's practice. In considering an individual case, each of these bodies has a narrower focus, usually confined to the care of a single patient. It is rare for an inquiry body to consider concurrently cases involving one doctor and several patients: if it does so, the inquirer must be careful not to allow evidence from one case to taint consideration of another case. Contrast this with the medical approach of seeking a full history and considering any similar episodes, before making a diagnosis.

Even when the focus of an inquiry body is the systems that allowed a problem doctor to continue practising (as was the case in my Tauranga Hospitals Inquiry),[126] the law may operate to constrain the ambit of review. There may be significant 'grey' material – such as incident reports and previous complaints or concerns suggesting that a doctor's performance was subpar – but a later review will usually consider only evidence of proven problems from the doctor's past that are directly relevant to the matter now at issue. Logical steps in an inquiry, such as the use of a single expert to advise on the quality of care for different patients, may give rise to an objection of potential bias.

It can be surprisingly difficult to uncover the full picture of a doctor's practice in court proceedings. If an injured patient's lawyer seeks to find out, from a surgeon or his or her employer, what that surgeon's rate of complications is for the type of operation in which the claimant patient was injured, discovery of the 'similar fact' information is likely to be resisted. In civil and criminal cases, the law generally excludes similar fact evidence unless its probative value outweighs its prejudicial effect.[127]

In exceptional cases judges will allow propensity evidence to be submitted,[128] but far more commonly it is excluded. Doctors may also be able to invoke the cloak of statutory protection available to information (such as complication rates) gathered as part of a 'protected quality assurance activity'.[129] Such protection is an explicit legislative trade-off to encourage health practitioners to engage in quality improvement activities without the fear that the resulting data will be used against them in legal proceedings.[130] It is doubtless a very good idea, although hard evidence of improvements as a result of such protection is difficult to find, despite requirements to provide the Minister of Health with annual reports, including information about how 'improvements in the competence or practice of the provider ... are to be monitored'.[131]

Silos of information

In practice it becomes extremely difficult to piece together all the evidence of competence concerns that may be held by various sources: an employer, a medical indemnity insurer, a compensation scheme or claims body such as the Accident Compensation Scheme in New Zealand or the National Health Service Litigation Authority in the United Kingdom, a medical board, or a health complaints commission or ombudsman.

The problem of silos of disconnected information about a health practitioner is a familiar one to health policy-makers and inquiry bodies, but attempts to solve it encounter implacable opposition from professional bodies. All too often, complaints and concerns about individual doctors are dealt with in isolation, in a reactive way that relies on patients/complainants or whistle-blowing colleagues; and the outcomes of complaint processes and external reviews about individual medical practice are shrouded in secrecy and not readily available to the public. The pieces of the jigsaw puzzle are not connected until late in the day.

In 2000, there was public concern in New Zealand about the slow handling of a serious complaint of negligence by a gynaecologist, and the possibility of a pattern of poor practice going undetected, despite pockets of data about this practitioner being held by separate statutory agencies. Up to 70 complaints were laid by Northland women against Dr Graham Parry. He was ultimately found guilty of disgraceful conduct in relation to one patient, Colleen Poutsma (who told her story to the media, as she lay dying), but exonerated in relation to the multiple other allegations.

As a judge said, the facts did not support 'the public's hue and cry'.[132] No pattern of poor practice was evident from the many complaints. In the aftermath of these events, Dr Parry was said to epitomise the risk that adverse media publicity may fuel unjustified complaints and unfairly tarnish the reputation of a good practitioner.[133] Yet the case also illustrates the limitations of legal processes that look at single complaints or concerns in isolation and apply differing tests for a compensation claim, a complaint inquiry, and a disciplinary prosecution. None constituted a full review or audit of the doctor's practice.

In response to public concern about the Poutsma case, the Minister of Health commissioned an inquiry into whether there were 'any regulatory and institutional barriers to information sharing and co-ordination regarding adverse medical outcomes' between three key statutory agencies: the Accident Compensation Corporation (ACC, handling claims from injured patients), the Health and Disability Commissioner (HDC, handling patient complaints), and the Medical Practitioners Disciplinary Tribunal (hearing charges of professional discipline against doctors). The inquiry report, *Review of Processes Concerning Adverse Medical Events*,[134] confirmed the existence of information silos that could allow poor practice to continue undetected.

Inquiry chair Helen Cull noted that the various agencies were not required to share information, and did not do so; and that '[w]ithout access to information about a practitioner on a centralised system, or any audit powers of an independent body, this becomes a barrier impeding a timely identification of adverse medical outcomes by medical practitioners'[135] and may lead to each agency dealing with the same practitioner in isolation. Cull concluded that the 'lack of a centralised information system, containing relevant information about accepted claims or proven complaints by a practitioner, impedes a timely identification of a practitioner whose practice is below acceptable standards',[136] and recommended the creation of a central database.

It is telling that, over a decade later, there is still no centralised database of information from claims, complaints and concerns about health practitioners in New Zealand.[137] Reforms did ensue from the Cull Inquiry, with enactment of the Health Practitioners Competence Assurance Act 2003 and the Health and Disability Commissioner Amendment Act 2003. One positive development is the requirement that key agencies share information. This has proved helpful between HDC and the registration boards since if, for example, it emerges that the Medical Council is already undertaking a performance assessment because of concerns about a doctor, HDC can forward any complaints about that doctor, to inform the Council's deliberations.

However, it takes a motivated patient or family to complain to HDC, or a brave colleague or employer to notify the Medical Council of concerns. As noted earlier, even following death or a serious adverse event, in fewer than 1 in 25 cases is a formal complaint made. One would expect a much larger pool of data of poor practice to be available from ACC, since the fairly low threshold for cover for 'treatment injury' means there are few disincentives to deter injured patients from claiming. Patients who suffer an unexpected complication from treatment are entitled to earnings compensation and rehabilitation, so one might expect a high claims rate. Yet, counterintuitively, the proportion of injured patients who make a treatment injury claim remains relatively low, very close to the proportion of claimants in tort (negligence) systems in the United States.[138]

In theory, claims data should reveal whether a particular service, and even an individual practitioner, has an unduly high rate of injury or complications, after adjusting for volume and complexity of patients. The legislative provisions authorising cover for treatment injury impose a specific obligation on ACC, if it believes, from information collected in the course of processing treatment injury claims, that there is 'a risk of harm to the public', to 'report the risk, and any other relevant information, to the authority responsible for patient safety in relation to the treatment that caused the personal injury'.[139] This means that ACC is required to report individual doctors to the Medical Council, and hospitals or medical centres to the Director-General of Health, if claims data indicates a risk of harm to the public arising from the work of that doctor or health facility.

David Studdert and Troy Brennan, experts in patient safety and the law, acknowledge that, in rare cases, patients are harmed by physicians who are 'incompetent, dangerous, or malevolent', and that even a no-fault compensation scheme 'must have mechanisms in place to deal with such practitioners, either directly or by triaging them to appropriate disciplinary bodies'.[140] Joanna Manning, explaining the New Zealand no-fault compensation scheme, notes that '[t]he public's memory of recent "health scandals" was sufficiently fresh that it was considered unacceptable for the ACC not to share concerns about individual practitioners or potential public safety issues identified through the claims process'.[141]

From a public viewpoint, it is inconceivable that a statutory claims agency could sit on information indicating a risk of harm to patients from an individual practitioner, without bringing the matter to the attention of the relevant registration board. This was one of the information silo problems highlighted in the Cull Inquiry, and the rationale for Parliament legislating for mandatory 'risk of harm' reporting as part of the new treatment injury provisions.

However, ACC's risk of harm reporting has not proven straightforward. The focus in assessing claims is simply on the nature of the treatment injury, and claims data is usually insufficiently detailed to determine the cause of a patient injury. Practitioner error may 'be "fudged" in the claims process, given entrenched professional reticence about error'.[142] It also seems probable that ACC's decisions (about whether the risk of harm threshold for reporting has been reached) are influenced by a natural reluctance to undermine practitioner willingness to assist injured patients make claims. After a strong reaction from the medical profession in the first year of reporting, when ACC made 30 reports to the Medical Council under the risk of harm provisions, the average number of reports has dropped to six per year in the past four years.[143] An 'information gap' has opened up in the new legislation,[144] and it may be difficult for ACC to conclude that a risk of harm exists, or to make a meaningful report about it.

Doctors and other practitioners are understandably wary of the consequences of risk of harm reports to registration boards, since they might trigger a board to undertake a review of their competence to practise. Fears of being reported to their registration board have been cited as a reason for health practitioner resistance to providing detailed treatment injury claims information to ACC. Since practitioner co-operation is essential in completing claim forms on behalf of injured patients, ACC is understandably nervous about undermining practitioner confidence in the treatment injury scheme.

As a consequence, ACC has made relatively few reports to registration boards under the mandatory risk reporting provisions. Comparative information at individual practitioner level is not available. Even at service level, hospitals and district health boards do not receive detailed information comparing their treatment injury rates for particular procedures with those of other hospitals or boards. The high hopes that ACC treatment injury data would be a catalyst for patient safety improvements[145] appear not to have been fully realised. To navigate these roadblocks, we need a roadmap.

From roadblocks to roadmap

In this part of the book, I have described the myriad players in the health system and their relevance to any discussion of medical competence. In various ways, they actively bolster or passively acquiesce in a system where the ongoing competence of doctors is not assured.

I have identified five main roadblocks to change: undemanding patients, overburdened doctors, reluctant regulators, medical culture, and legal constraints. The forces that support the status quo are well embedded. Cultural factors are deep-seated and resistant to change. But changes are occurring internationally. Some governments, professional societies and regulators are grasping the nettle to require better information for patients and robust checks on doctors' competence, incorporating feedback from patients and colleagues. If successfully implemented, these changes have the potential to ensure that patients encounter only 'good doctors' and to underpin a new medical professionalism.

In the final part, I present a prescription for change.

4

PRESCRIPTION FOR CHANGE
WHAT CAN WE IMPROVE?

I started this book with a simple proposition: in an ideal world, we would know that every licensed doctor is a competent doctor – that he or she meets the minimum standards of being a good doctor. Our health and regulatory systems would provide us with that assurance. As members of the public, and potential patients, we would be able to rely on the fact that someone is listed on the public medical register and has a current licence to practise medicine as assurance that doctor is competent.

In this final part of the book, I make some suggestions to improve the current state of affairs: a prescription for change. My focus is on three main areas where I see the most pressing need for improvement: information for patients; recertification of doctors; and public trust in the medical profession. These topics and my recommendations are closely interrelated. The changes I suggest are practical and achievable. If implemented, my recommendations will help solve many of the problems described in this book. They aim to support, not undermine, professionalism, and to give patients justified reassurance.

Better information for patients, from trusted sources, will give people more confidence when they seek medical care. Enhanced recertification processes will help reassure the public and support doctors in their own efforts to keep up to date and meet patient expectations. Firm regulators (with greater lay membership) that are proactive in checking competence, rigorous in responding to notified concerns, and open about their work, will provide visible evidence of an effective safety net around medical practice. Together, these changes should help build public trust in the medical profession.

In making the case for change, I point to evidence from countries where good progress is being made in ensuring medical competence and publishing useful quality information for patients and the public: notably the United Kingdom, the United States and Canada. The cardiothoracic surgeons of Great Britain have shown the way, with their approach of 'modern medical professionalism'.[1] The American Board of Internal

Medicine has developed sophisticated quality improvement tools to bring the maintenance of medical competence into the twenty-first century. Medical regulators in Canada and the General Medical Council in the United Kingdom have shown a commitment to protecting the public by ensuring proper standards in the practice of medicine. My recommendations have particular relevance for New Zealand and Australia, where similar changes are overdue.

Summary so far

To recap, we've seen that patients expect their doctor to be competent, to have maintained their skills, and to be up to date in their medical knowledge. They also want their doctor to have effective communication skills and be able to establish a good relationship with them as a patient. In terms of personal qualities, patients expect their doctors to have integrity and be trustworthy, and to show a respectful, caring attitude. These attributes are mirrored in doctors' own expectations of what makes a good doctor. Patients also expect the relevant authorities to make proper checks to ensure doctors remain competent and fit to practise – and assume that this already occurs.

By and large, patients' expectations of their doctor are fulfilled. Most doctors do maintain their competence and perform at a good level, because they are self-motivated to do so and see it as a professional obligation. The most common problems patients encounter are poor communication skills and inadequate record-keeping, rather than deficits in knowledge or skill. Complaints about lack of respect and an uncaring attitude are also fairly common, though not confined to doctors.

Patients generally report high levels of trust in their individual doctor, although the medical profession as a whole scores less highly for trustworthiness. Research undertaken for the New Zealand Medical Council in 2007 shows relatively low levels of trust in doctors amongst the New Zealand public.² Only 9 per cent of the public thought that doctors in general were 'very trustworthy', compared with 43 per cent holding that opinion of their own doctor; 7 per cent of respondents thought their own doctor 'very untrustworthy'! These levels of trust appear to be lower than comparable surveys conducted in other countries.³

Patients routinely experience frustrating problems when they seek medical care. It's difficult for people to obtain meaningful information about doctors. Finding a new doctor is hard enough; obtaining basic information, let alone comparative quality information, about a prospective doctor is very difficult. Patients have to take it on trust that their doctor is a good doctor. Probably around 5 per cent of doctors are practising poorly (below the threshold of good medical practice), and 2 per cent may pose a threat to patient safety. At present, patients cannot confidently rely on medical professionalism or regulatory oversight to ensure good medical practice. In a survey for the New Zealand Medical Council in 2010, 75 per cent of respondents said their confidence in doctors would be increased if they knew that doctors' performance was subject to a regular review.⁴

The problems described in this book are not new, but they have proven fairly intractable in many countries for decades. We've seen the roadblocks that preserve the status quo. From amongst the large cast of players, I identified undemanding patients, overburdened doctors and reluctant regulators as contributing to an unsatisfactory situation. Their impact is amplified by ingrained medical culture and legal constraints. These are the factors that must be overcome if change is to be achieved.

Modest reforms have begun to surface in various jurisdictions, usually driven by political response to a medical scandal. Professional resistance has been vigorous and effective, although a few professional champions of reform have emerged. How, then, to approach further reform? If change is to be implemented successfully in the future, it must be consistent with well-established patient expectations, have political backing, and be seen by doctors themselves as fair, proportionate and workable.

Busy doctors will need to be persuaded of the rationale for any changes (that there will be benefits for patients *and* doctors) and confident that any new requirements will not be burdensome, time-consuming and expensive. Martin Marshall aptly notes of revalidation proposals in the United Kingdom that '[o]ver the years, doctors have proved themselves highly able to deal with bureaucracy, going through the motions, ticking the right boxes and getting on with what they regard as really important'.[5]

In seeking the optimal balance between professionalism and external regulation, the solution is likely to be found in a model of professionally supported regulation that fulfils the expectations of the public without undermining the self-motivation of individual doctors – what Marshall calls 'integrating regulatory and educational approaches to improvement'.[6] Cyril Chantler also makes this point powerfully:

> It is perhaps better for physicians as well as for society that physicians should work for love as well as for money and that they should protect their own professionalism. Physicians need trust more than regulation, but it is up to them to introduce systems that are comprehensive and fit for most purposes but not too bureaucratic and burdensome.[7]

If doctors lose their professional motivation at a time when many are already finding medical practice burdensome, all the best-laid recertification plans in the world will be for naught. As noted in the 2011 United Kingdom White Paper *Enabling Excellence*: 'The vast majority of healthcare workers ... do not strive to provide excellent care because they fear regulatory action if they do wrong or because they are told to do things properly. They do so because they are caring people, who are well trained and well motivated.'[8]

Doctors want regulation to be light-handed, but patients want it to be demonstrably effective. The challenge is to find that balance. I believe in the goodwill and motivation of medical practitioners to be 'good doctors', but in my view the profession and its regulators need a firm nudge in the right direction. Promising changes are occurring internationally in the availability of accessible information for patients, and in periodic checks of doctors' competence. They signpost the way forward.

Better information for patients

People seeking to access medical care (especially when facing a health crisis) often need help to find a doctor. At general practice level, prospective patients want basic information about a doctor, including whether he or she has the appropriate skills and qualifications to meet their health needs. They want to be confident their practitioner will be a good doctor. Ideally, they want a recommendation from a reliable source to help them make a choice, assuming there's one to be made. When referred to hospital or a secondary care specialist, patients want the same things, but they will hopefully get a helpful pointer from their general practitioner, if they have one.

Why should we try to meet patients' occasional need for information? We've seen that patients are fairly complacent about the lack of information currently available about how to find a doctor, how doctors compare, and how they can be confident that any licensed doctor will be competent. There's little evidence of people clamouring for this kind of information, even though the health sector is lagging behind other information-rich service areas. Why not concentrate on ensuring that doctor recertification processes are rigorous, so that patients can be confident that every licensed doctor is a good doctor?

Better information for patients and enhanced recertification processes are not mutually exclusive. There are several good reasons for improving the availability of healthcare quality information for patients and the public. That information may be about the quality of individual doctors, where reliable data at doctor level can be generated. More likely, the information will compare the quality of health services in which doctors work. The arguments that follow support the availability of both kinds of comparative information.

First, if medical ethics and law so highly value patient autonomy and choice in relation to informed consent to medical treatment, why deprive people of the information they need to make a prior (and possibly more significant) decision about their choice of doctor or health service? If the answer is that reliable information simply doesn't exist, shouldn't that be rectified? The ethical principle of respect for autonomy supports the case for the availability of information about doctors as well as about treatment options.

Secondly, the generation and supply of information to the public ought to be one way in which the medical profession holds itself accountable to the community. Governments invest significant amounts of funding in training the medical workforce, and registration as a doctor confers privileges on the practitioner. Part of the *quid pro quo*, particularly when the profession still enjoys a fair degree of autonomy in regulating itself, is to demand clear evidence of standards being maintained. This is an obvious form of accountability, and transparency (of the processes to maintain standards and the outcomes of those processes) provides evidence that words are being backed by action.

Finally, there is a cogent quality improvement argument for publication of information. Even if consumers' use of comparative information about the quality of doctors and health services is sporadic, doctors and healthcare organisations themselves are (or should be) interested in this sort of information. There is good research evidence that collating and publishing risk-adjusted data on key indicators will lead to improvements in quality.[9] It's hardly surprising that high-performing individuals like doctors and healthcare organisations (comprised of clinicians and managers) are motivated to learn from better-performing individuals and groups, and to lift their game. The competitive urge to improve performance is well ingrained in health as in other industries, and publication of information can be a spur to improvement.

So, arguments based on respect for autonomy, accountability, and quality improvement support the case for making comparative health quality information available to the public.[10] I am not here arguing for the proliferation of doctor-rating websites and magazines found in the United States, where the Zagat Survey company, better known for its popular restaurant guides, now produces a guide to doctors. As historian Nancy Tomes notes, the deluge of health consumer oriented information in the United States 'is an approach to health care choice rooted in the needs of affluent Americans with the financial and educational resources required to "shop" for care'. The end result is 'a complicated, chaotic, potentially toxic information environment'.[11] However, that does not detract from the utility of doctor report cards produced by government agencies or professional societies. Reputable reports from reliable sources can provide evidence and public assurance that a doctor or health service is performing to a good standard.

What about negative information concerning doctors who have been subject to adverse rulings in official complaint investigations or disciplinary hearings, or to malpractice settlements or awards or paid compensation claims? There is debate about the significance of such information and whether or not it is a marker of incompetence. After all, compared with feedback surveys from multiple patients, or report cards aggregating data from multiple procedures, complaint and disciplinary findings and malpractice or compensation claims are usually confined to single episodes of care. Many doctors dispute the relevance of this sort of information, and regard its disclosure as an unwarranted invasion of their privacy. Yet a moment's reflection suggests that, if they have a choice of doctor, prospective patients are likely to be interested in finding out about even individual instances of complaints, discipline, malpractice and compensation payouts. This is precisely why defence lawyers typically fight so hard to suppress such information, to protect the doctor's reputation.

Most complaint and disciplinary information, claims data and malpractice settlements entered by insurers on a doctor's behalf have traditionally been hidden from public view behind a veil of secrecy.[12] Doctors are very rarely named following investigations by official complaint agencies, and sometimes obtain name suppression even after being found guilty of a disciplinary offence. The situation falls short of what Judge Silvia Cartwright envisaged when making the case for an independent medical complaints and disciplinary system in New Zealand: 'The vast majority [of patients] want information . . . and *the right to ensure that a negligent, rude or incompetent doctor's reputation is known* so that other patients can choose alternative health care.'[13]

Secrecy risks undermining public confidence in the health professions and disciplinary procedures. As Health and Disability Commissioner, I noted: 'The public is currently being "kept in the dark" about information that may influence a person's choice of practitioner or facility, and there is an increasing public desire for openness. More than a decade after the public disquiet that led to the overhaul of the complaints and medical disciplinary system, it is still common to read headlines like "Outrage at 'old boys' network that protects medics".'[14]

However, a balance needs to be drawn between the legitimate privacy interests of doctors, and the public interest. I question the fairness or value of naming doctors about whom complaints are upheld, unless there is a public safety reason to do so or the doctor is a 'frequent flier'. The policy instituted during my time as Commissioner adopts this approach.[15] One swallow (or even two) does not a summer make, and it always struck me as disproportionate to put a doctor's reputation on the line on the basis of limited complaint information. But a doctor should be publicly named if there is a risk of harm to patients or the doctor's track record justifies naming. If the doctor's complaint or claims history shows a pattern of substandard care or communication, indicating an underlying problem, that *is* the sort of information patients would want to know about – and in my view should be entitled to access.

Similarly, medical disciplinary findings should not be suppressed – especially in an era when only the most serious cases go to discipline. Increasingly, discipline is reserved for unethical conduct (such as sexual or financial exploitation of patients) or reckless or grossly negligent clinical care. Public confidence in the accountability processes for medical discipline requires that guilty doctors be named. Name suppression should be reserved for truly exceptional circumstances, such as to preserve the confidentiality of a patient who could otherwise be identified. Disciplinary tribunals effectively function as health courts, and are a remnant of the privilege of self-regulation. Justice in the regular courts is overwhelmingly public and open. So, too, the meting out of discipline in professional tribunals should be transparent, consistent with accountability to the public rather than the profession.

In the New Zealand context, the case for open discipline is well made by Joanna Manning:

> Indeed, there is a strong argument that the principles of open justice and reporting weigh even more heavily in respect of professional disciplinary tribunals in the health field than for criminal courts. The reason is that there are so few avenues in New Zealand for the public airing of health and disability complaints, given the absence of medical malpractice actions and the existence of confidential compensation and complaints systems.[16]

One final point is that where doctors *are* named following disciplinary processes, medical regulators should make it easy for members of the public to search a doctor's history and find adverse findings that are in the public domain.[17]

What about malpractice claims data (held by insurers or agencies such as the National Health Service Litigation Authority (NHSLA) in the United Kingdom) and treatment injury claims data in countries like New Zealand, with state compensation schemes for medical (and other) accidents? This information is, like much complaints information, currently shielded from the public and even from medical regulators. Yet it may well be a marker of incompetence, especially if there is a pattern of behaviour leading to settled or paid claims. In the United States, malpractice settlements and awards are reported to the National Practitioner Data Bank,[18] where the information is available to state medical boards, hospitals and insurers. However, where the NHSLA handles a negligence claim and identifies poor performance by an individual doctor, the General Medical Council is not notified; instead, the concerns are followed up directly with the NHS employer.[19] When medical defence insurers in the United Kingdom and Australia settle claims on behalf of doctors, the GMC or Medical Board of Australia is not notified.[20]

The New Zealand and Scandinavian compensation schemes for injured patients do not make claims information about practitioners or facilities publicly available. I recall the explanation given by the head of the Danish compensation scheme for the quarantine over claims data about individual doctors: 'That is the price we pay for the doctors' co-operation.'[21] Michelle Mello and colleagues, analysing the New Zealand and Scandinavian patient compensation schemes, note that '[a] perceived advantage of the information firewall is that it encourages physicians to make patients aware of their right to seek compensation and to assist them in claiming, which physicians might be reluctant to do if they feared a compensation claim could trigger or facilitate disciplinary action'.[22]

The point of sharing such information is not to prompt discipline – there are other pathways for that. The reason for notifying a medical board that claims information shows an individual doctor may pose a risk of harm to patients is to enable the board to assess whether a review of that doctor's practice is warranted. It is not sufficient to wait for a patient, colleague or employer to lodge a concern with a medical board. Agencies handling complaints or malpractice or compensation claims should have a low threshold for alerting the regulator where there is evidence of a pattern of concerning medical behaviour.

During my time as Health and Disability Commissioner, we erred on the side of sharing information with the regulator, in the face of vigorous opposition from the aptly named Medical Protection Society. We signed an information-sharing memorandum of understanding with the Medical Council, agreeing to notify the Council when HDC 'is aware of three or more similar "low level" matters relating to a registered medical practitioner within the past five years, which may indicate a pattern of conduct indicative of wider competence concerns'.[23] The purpose was to ensure that frequent fliers did not fly under the radar. A small group of doctors are often subject to a disproportionate number of complaints.[24] If a doctor is an outlier by attracting several complaints – even if they do not proceed to formal investigation and a breach finding – that is likely to be a pointer to problems in their practice that warrant closer scrutiny by the regulator. Having a low threshold for alerting the regulator is especially important when the complaint agency favours 'low level resolution' by informal means, and does not formally investigate most complaints.[25]

I doubt that members of the public want to delve into a doctor's complaints or claims history. But patients would expect their medical regulator to be appraised of all relevant information about a doctor's standard of practice and take it into account when issuing annual licences or practising certificates. I suspect members of the public would be surprised to know how much subterranean information (about complaints, malpractice claims and compensation claims) never sees the light of day in the offices of a medical board. These agencies, charged with ensuring doctors are competent, are not playing with a full deck of cards. They need more information, to better protect the public.

What patients find when looking for information
It's difficult to generalise about the information available to patients in different countries. Commonly, it's hard to find a doctor in the first place.

Even in the United States, the respected Consumer Health Reports tells website readers, 'finding the right doctor for you involves cobbling together information from a variety of sources, including your own observations and interactions with your doctor'.[26] There are thousands of sources of information about physicians in North America on the internet, but the quality and accuracy of that information is highly variable.[27]

If, having found a doctor, you want to dig a little deeper, you will struggle to find useful information about their credentials. Some comparative quality information is published in the United Kingdom and the United States (mainly comparing hospitals, but in some cases at the level of individual surgeons), but very little in Australia and New Zealand. And with a few exceptions, medical regulators in all countries do a mediocre job of providing a full picture of a doctor's practice profile.

Patients looking for a doctor in New Zealand have no easy way to do so. If you type 'find a doctor in New Zealand' into Google, a fairly random list of websites appears: some commercial, and none very helpful. The Ministry of Health's website, under the heading 'Choosing your GP', tells readers that, in New Zealand, 'you can choose the doctor or medical centre that you visit'[28] – but then simply refers to the Medical Council register and to district health board websites that are difficult to navigate and, in most cases, contain very little information about individual doctors. Other sites refer readers to the white pages of the telephone book, for a list of general practices in the area. This is about as good as it gets.

Let's assume you find the name of a doctor and want to get some independent information about them and their practice. The logical place to search is the website of the regulator, the New Zealand Medical Council (www.mcnz.org.nz), though many people are unaware of the Council's role. The information under 'Find a Registered Doctor' on the Council's website allows the reader to search by the doctor's surname, but is limited to their date of graduation, practice district, whether they hold a current practising certificate, scope of practice, and conditions (if any) on their practice. The reason for the imposition of any conditions is not disclosed. If you want to know whether the doctor has been found guilty of a disciplinary offence, you need to go to a separate website (www.hpdt.org.nz) and know where to search by name (and for their pre-2004 disciplinary history, you need to search a different website). The Medical Council recognises that there should be a direct link from an individual doctor's entry on the online register to any disciplinary tribunal adverse findings,[29] but has not yet facilitated this. In the meantime, searching the register is not an exercise for the faint-hearted.

Nor is it much easier in other countries. A Toronto *Globe and Mail* article in 2011 advised readers wanting to do a background check on a doctor to consult the website of the provincial college of physicians and surgeons body (the medical regulator in Canada), but found that many colleges make it difficult to trace disciplinary history.[30] A notable exception is the College of Physicians and Surgeons of Ontario, where a simple 'Doctor Search' function on the home page enables an easy search of the doctor's registration history and practice location, and provides full details of any disciplinary findings and even court findings of professional negligence.

In the United States, the Federation of State Medical Boards, on payment of a $9.95 fee, provides members of the public with a 'DocInfo Profile' for a named physician, listing qualifications, board certification status, state(s) where licensed, and disciplinary history. At least 22 states have passed laws requiring that medical boards provide basic physician profiles on their websites, but links to disciplinary findings are variable.[31] There is also the National Practitioner Data Bank, created by Congress in 1986, which records physicians' disciplinary findings and malpractice settlements and awards, but the information is available only to state medical boards, hospitals and insurers. The Obama administration shut down the public use section of the website in September 2011 because of physician privacy concerns, even though the data in that section is anonymised.[32]

Registration boards should make full information about registered practitioners easily accessible, but few present a user-friendly face to the public, at least via their websites. A review of the relevant New Zealand legislation noted the lack of website information that is 'clearly written for the public or users of health services', and recommended that boards make information about registered practitioners freely available.[33] The Midwifery Council website is better than most.[34] It provides a link on its home page to midwives who are suspended or have been removed from the register. It also has a link to advice on 'How to find a midwife', with some practical suggestions for consumers. But this example is the exception, not the rule.

The other sort of official information that is often held centrally but not always shared with clinicians, let alone the public, is outcomes data gathered as part of hospital episode statistics.[35] As Ian Kennedy famously observed in his inquiry report, Bristol Royal Infirmary was 'awash with data', but no one was analysing it.[36] Investigative journalists have on occasion invoked freedom of information legislation to great effect, to compel disclosure of health data in the public interest. The newspaper *Newsday* used this tactic successfully in New York in 1990, to obtain and publish surgeon-specific cardiac mortality data. The *Guardian* newspaper used freedom of information laws to obtain and publish similar data about cardiac surgeons in the northwest of England in 2005. In both cases the public interest in disclosure was seen to override any privacy concerns – even though the information enabled comparisons of individual doctors. In New Zealand, the media has not yet been so adventurous, confining official information requests to health board data.[37]

Information about a doctor's track record in New Zealand – for example, rate of complications for a specific procedure, the outcomes of employer credentialling processes[38] or Medical Council competence reviews, and complaints, disciplinary and claims history – is currently shielded from public view. The shroud of secrecy surrounding sensitive information around doctors' performance (and health service performance in general) is remarkable, as the following example demonstrates.

Quality assurance – a case study in secrecy
Like many countries, New Zealand has passed legislation to protect from disclosure any activities 'undertaken to improve the practices or competence of 1 or more health practitioners by assessing the health services performed by those practitioners'.[39] The protection conferred means that clinicians who apply for such cover can review their work with a view to improvement, in the knowledge that any information generated cannot be disclosed to a third party or in a judicial proceeding or investigation. In return for this statutory privilege, persons responsible for the activity are required to file with the Minister of Health reports about 'improvements in the competence or practice of the provider' resulting from such activities – a form of accountability to check that improvements are actually being made.[40] Might not the public be entitled to learn, from these reports, what kinds of improvements have been generated, particularly when the statute authorises the release of non-identifying information?[41] No, says the timorous Ministry of Health, claiming that to disclose it (even without identifiers) would prejudice the future supply of such information.[42] This denial could be challenged by going to the Ombudsman, invoking the statutory principle that official information 'shall be made available unless there is good reason for withholding it'.[43] But why should it be necessary to go to such lengths to obtain basic health information about clinical quality?

Where else might members of the public look for information about doctors? One obvious place is organisations that employ doctors. But here, too, the published information is sparse. The primary health organisations and district health boards who employ doctors in the New Zealand publicly funded health system make very limited information about clinicians available to their communities. A few health boards list on their website (though it requires a diligent search) the senior doctors working in a hospital by service, with details of qualifications, registration status and specialty area. (Some even manage a photo!) The majority of boards publish lots of information about their own governance and structure, but no details about the consultants who will be responsible for the patient's care. The inquiring patient referred to hospital and wanting to glean some basic information about their specialist will find it difficult to do so. (Much more information about specialists is found on private hospital websites, reflecting the competitive market for business.)

Admittedly, patients have very little choice of doctor at a public hospital. New Zealand law gives them the right 'to express a preference as to who will provide services and have that preference met where practicable',[44] but in practice it is seldom practicable to meet patient preferences for a particular hospital consultant. It should nonetheless be standard practice to publish information about the senior doctors working in hospital services, with details of their qualifications, registration and credentialled status, and specialty area. Patients might also be reassured if hospitals clearly identified (on their website) the steps taken to credential all employed doctors, even if employers shy away from publishing qualitative information about staff.

Funders of health care in New Zealand and Australia have been reluctant to use the lever of mandatory publication of healthcare quality information comparing the performance of publicly funded organisations such as hospitals – let alone compel disclosure of information at practitioner level. It may be that the data currently collected is not of consistent or sufficient quality to enable meaningful comparisons. Governments may be anxious to avoid picking a fight with powerful medical associations that would challenge any moves in this direction as 'naming, shaming and blaming'. They may also be nervous about exposing the poor performance of hospitals and igniting community concern, which may have electoral consequences in an area as politically sensitive as publicly funded health care.

Given the relatively limited policy levers available to governments as funders of health care, in seeking to improve quality and ensure good value for public funding, the failure to use the lever of transparency of information is remarkable. Only in more recent times have governments in New Zealand (tentatively, for areas such as wait times for cancer treatment or elective surgery) and Australia (more ambitiously, with its new MyHospitals website)[45] started to follow Northern Hemisphere moves in this direction, at least for district health board or hospital performance. Queensland Health has been the most innovative, using statistical process control measures to compare public hospital performance, with public reporting of improvement actions taken by outlier hospitals. It is telling that this initiative has occurred in the state most deeply shaken by a health scandal (Bundaberg Hospital and Dr Patel).[46] Does the public have to wait for a scandal to provoke greater transparency about health system performance?

My information prescription[47]

So, what are my specific recommendations to enable patients to get better information about how to find a doctor, and information about a doctor's credentials and track record? My recommendations are aimed at health systems that are predominantly publicly funded.

The first three recommendations are relatively straightforward – they are not threatening, and simply require basic information to be made easily accessible for patients. The fourth recommendation, relating to collation and publication of comparative healthcare quality data, presents a much greater challenge, but has the potential to better inform the community and improve health care.

1. Publicly funded local health organisations should be required to publish easily accessible information about how to find a primary care doctor in their locality. Patients need details of the name, qualifications, registration status and specialty area of all doctors working

in their local community, and whether or not they are admitting new patients. Funders should, by contract or regulation, require the publication of up-to-date information along these lines. The aim is simply to make it easier for patients to find basic information about how to access medical care. Similar information should ideally be available about medical specialists in private practice in the community, but the market and general practitioner recommendations should adequately cater for that need.

2. Medical regulators should be encouraged (by firm directives from Ministers of Health or Health Select Committees, if necessary) to provide a 'doctor search' function on their website, facilitating an easy check of a doctor's registration status, registration history, specialist certification (if any), currency of practising certificate, restrictions (if any) on practice (with an explanation of the reasons), practice location, and full details of any disciplinary findings that are not suppressed (with links to relevant decisions). The aim here is to enable members of the public to have one central place where they can obtain up-to-date registration status information, as well as negative information that some prospective patients will want to be aware of. Providing such information is an important way for regulators to be transparent and accountable to the public they are charged with protecting.

3. Employers should publish details of the senior doctors working in hospital services, with details of their qualifications, registration and credentialled status, and specialty area – and spell out the steps taken to credential those doctors. Private hospitals should publish the same information about the specialists to whom they grant visiting privileges. To make this happen, funding agreements should require the publication of such information and health system regulators should make it a requirement for accreditation of hospital facilities.

The rationale is to meet the basic information needs of patients and to give some reassurance of the steps taken to credential all employed or visiting doctors, even if the hospital or primary care trust shies away from publishing qualitative information about medical staff. In the competitive private hospital market, it is surprising that leading institutions are not already making such information freely available. In the public system, where patients in most countries have few choices, funders and accreditation agencies need to ensure this information gap is filled.

4. Medical colleges and specialty societies should follow the example of the Society for Cardiothoracic Surgery of Great Britain & Ireland (SCTS) and collect, analyse and publish data showing the quality of care provided by practitioner members. This would demonstrate to the public that the relevant group has set clear service standards and is committed to quality assurance and quality improvement. It would also be visible demonstration of a commitment to modern medical professionalism. Governments, using regulatory powers and providing funding and technical support, should require the collation of agreed sets of healthcare quality data at hospital level and in primary care, and set a time frame for publication. In the short term, the aim should be to develop robust data comparing identified hospitals or teams with each other on quality indicators that clinicians agree are meaningful; in the medium term, that information should be made public; and in the long term (within a decade), data at individual clinician level should be shared, and then published. This is a radical but achievable information prescription, with the potential for significant quality gains.

Lessons from cardiac surgery
The history of the collection of clinical outcomes data by the cardiac surgical community is well documented.[48] Solid evidence has emerged that

the publication of surgeon-specific cardiac outcomes data has not simply fuelled media curiosity. It has benefited patients. A 40 per cent reduction in risk-adjusted mortality has been reported in the United States[49] and the United Kingdom[50] following the introduction of public reporting of results, and this has been achieved without denying surgery to high-risk patients. These are compelling results. Although the mechanism and quantum of improvement remains contentious, the positive impact from well-designed public reporting programmes is clear.[51] In the words of SCTS President David Taggart: 'Nothing stimulates change like clear comparable and publicly accessible evidence.'[52]

A key point about the cardiac surgeons' initiative is that it was motivated by scientific inquiry – a quest to find out how many patients were dying in hospital from cardiac surgery, and to understand the reasons for any variations. In the 1990s, their data collection became more comprehensive (with most NHS hospitals participating) and reliable, using sophisticated risk-adjustment methods. The Bristol paediatric cardiac surgery inquiry was clearly a spur, but the key driver was the surgeons themselves, under the leadership of Bruce Keogh, who takes an uncompromising stance: 'Surgeons have a moral and professional duty to know what they are doing, how well they are doing it and to use that information to help them improve – otherwise they have no right to be doing it at all.'[53] This is a clear example of professionalism, rather than regulation, driving quality assurance and improvement.

Observers of the cardiac surgeons' journey have noted that culture was key – a surgical unit needed to have a strong desire to collate and analyse data – and that open publication of surgical results was the final stimulus. There was initially strong resistance from some surgeons who described the experience of 'media attack' following public reporting, noting that '[t]alented, hard working, and dedicated healthcare professionals were inappropriately forced to defend their practice' (by definition, 50 per cent of surgical units fall below the mean) and '[p]rospective patients and relatives were filled with unnecessary anxiety'.[54]

'League tables' has become a pejorative term, often used as code for damaging comparisons that lack validity but are used to damn below-average performers. The controversy over the public release of league tables comparing the academic success of schools, and the vehement resistance from teachers, highlights some of the tensions. Obviously the data needs to be fairly robust – although it is also important to make a start, and not let 'the perfect be the enemy of the good'.[55] There are inevitably risks of sensationalist media reporting, scapegoating and perverse effects. But if the data that underpins the league tables is robust and the quality indicators chosen are important for patient outcomes, and educative for providers, there is a strong case for using the lever of publication to inform and improve. As Marshall and colleagues note, '[p]ublic reports are here to stay, and the debate should now be moving on from whether to use them to how best to deploy them in particular circumstances'.[56]

Naturally, in the early days, some surgeons were apprehensive about being identified as poor performers. Critical to the acceptance of open reporting of outcomes was having clear, agreed principles for explaining divergence. Many 'abnormal' outcomes will turn out on further investigation to be due to normal variation. Detection of unexpected variance should trigger further investigation, but not precipitate action against a surgeon or unit. Better data collection, analysis and follow-up has led to the detection of potential problems at an earlier stage, but fewer suspensions or restrictions.[57] So the cardiac surgeons' initiative turns out to be good for patients *and* doctors.

Unlike the first three recommendations, this one may take several years to lead to published information for patients. As noted by Bridgewater, '[t]he information available for patients undergoing orthopaedic surgery, upper gastrointestinal surgery, interventional cardiology procedures, and pretty much every other area of medicine also lags significantly behind cardiac surgery'.[58] In some surgical areas (such as vascular, orthopaedic and colo-rectal surgery), there is no reason why appropriate indicators could not be agreed fairly quickly, although the process of risk adjustment will inevitably take longer (as noted, it took the cardiac surgeons several years to develop statistically valid risk-adjustment criteria). In other specialties, such as internal medicine, psychiatry, obstetrics and general practice, it is likely to take longer to agree on relevant quality indicators that can be measured and reported on. But that is not a good reason not to make a start.

The first step is for the specialty groups to start collecting, analysing and sharing their own data. A few groups already do so. Valuable registries and databases currently exist.[59] The Australian and New Zealand Dialysis and Transplant Registry, which has collected dialysis and transplant data since 1977, with 100 per cent of renal units participating, is one example. It includes comparisons of units on key quality measures (peritonitis and access at first haemodialysis) related to patient mortality.[60] Units can see their own data and where they sit on a graph, but they are not able to identify other units, which means the data is not being used to its full potential for quality improvement purposes.

I recall attending a meeting of New Zealand health sector leaders with international quality guru Don Berwick,[61] when nervousness was expressed about sharing comparative data identifying district health boards amongst the boards. As Berwick asked: 'How are you going to learn from each other if you can't find out who's performing well?' Clinicians and units need to have the confidence to share identifying comparative quality data with each other. If cardiac surgeons can 'go public' with the most sensitive data – death rates – other groups should at least be able to begin sharing data openly with each other.

But in some areas, data is not uniformly collected, analysed or shared, even within specialty groups. A major *Guardian* newspaper investigation in England in 2010 examined death rates from planned vascular surgery for abdominal aortic aneurysm at 116 hospitals (using data obtained under freedom of information laws) and found a 'massive variation', with unacceptably high mortality in some hospitals. The *Guardian* trenchantly observed that '[d]octors in the NHS do not know how well they are performing and whether they are more likely than their colleagues to kill or cure their patients, because of a widespread failure to collect the information'.[62]

Since my recommendation is addressed to professional groups, it is an agenda that can only be driven effectively by clinicians. This has been called the professionally oriented model of public release of performance data.[63] Cardiac surgeon Ben Bridgewater, a leading figure in the efforts of the United Kingdom cardiac surgeons, has observed: 'The profession needs to furnish a public appetite for information. Some of that will inevitably be comparable information and to continue to maintain patients' trust in this era, putting some transparency and accountability systems in place are essential.'[64] Patient representatives have been strongly supportive of this approach: 'The whole medical profession must respond to these issues – sooner or later the public will demand it.'[65] It is time for other specialty groups to respond to the challenge of the cardiac surgeons.

Professionalism may need to be backed by governments using regulatory levers and providing funding support. The systems regulator, the Care Quality Commission (CQC), and the Department of Health work closely with the SCTS in overseeing the national cardiac surgery audit in England. All NHS hospitals are required to submit data; the CQC publishes risk-adjusted comparative data on its website, and the results feed into the star rating system for hospital trusts. The United Kingdom Department of Health is investing heavily in national clinical audits to extend transparency to other surgical specialties.[66]

Similar opportunities exist in Australia and New Zealand. The Royal Australasian College of Surgeons has overseen a voluntary audit of surgical mortality, begun in Western Australia and modelled on the Scottish audit of surgical mortality.[67] It has been embraced by all Australian states and territories (with funding support) and led to publication of an Australian audit of surgical mortality, identifying areas for improvement (e.g., prophylaxis to prevent deep vein thrombosis, and earlier transfer to

ICU).[68] The approach is educational, with all surgical Fellows required to participate as part of College continuing professional development requirements. However, the comparisons are high-level (by state, not individual hospital, let alone individual surgeon) and even then the states are not identified. There is obviously a long way to go before Australasian surgeons are ready to follow the lead of their British counterparts.

New Zealand is conspicuously absent from the so-called *Australian and New Zealand Audit of Surgical Mortality*, prompting audit chair Guy Maddern to say: 'There is hope that it can be further introduced into New Zealand; however, this has proven to be a greater challenge and it will perhaps take several more years until the New Zealand Ministry of Health recognizes the importance of the data being provided.'[69] I recall my dismay when New Zealand was the only country without reported data for surgical mortality (in contrast to the United States, Canada, United Kingdom, Netherlands, Germany and Australia) when OECD data was presented at a Commonwealth Fund international symposium on healthcare policy in Washington DC in November 2007.[70] It is high time this health information gap in New Zealand was rectified, with leadership from medical groups, and a spur from government.[71]

Nor should the publication of comparative data be confined to hospital-level services. Since most health care is delivered in the community, there is scope for funders to promote quality improvement, and provide useful information to the public, about the performance of local primary health organisations (PHOs) and their constituent general practices. As one district health board chief executive said to me: 'I could tell you which are the best-performing and worst-performing general practices in this district.'[72] If a public funder is sitting on that information, why shouldn't it be published? Not to punish, but to inform the community and to improve the quality of primary care. Yet, to date, very limited information about the performance of PHOs has been published in New Zealand. The published data has been confined to high-level process measures (such as the percentage of eligible patients offered a cervical smear or diabetic patients having an annual review and update of care plan).[73] Over time, comparative quality information across a wider range of indicators (that patients and doctors agree are important) should become publicly available not only at PHO level but also at the level of individual general practices.

Defining quality indicators in primary care is complex,[74] given the wide range of health conditions of presenting patients, the fact that care is often delivered in teams in which the doctor is only one player, and the multiple factors impacting on patient outcomes. The contribution of the individual general practitioner in patient care, compared with the surgeon performing an operation, is difficult to assess. However, a recent independent inquiry into the quality of general practice in the United Kingdom confirmed that 'important dimensions of quality of care in general practice can be measured, and routine data sets used, to assess the comparative performance of practices'.[75] The inquiry report noted that 'some aspects of an individual's performance can be assessed at the GP level through local audit and monitoring such as patient feedback, length and quality of consultation, accuracy of diagnosis and appropriateness of prescribing. Where possible, practices that commit to transparency in the publication of this kind of data would move towards greater public accountability.'[76]

The National Health Service in England is proceeding down this path as part of a government push for increased transparency.[77] The Department of Health plans to publish 'scorecards' rating the performance of GP practices against quality indicators, such as immunisation data and prescribing information. The proposal drew a curious response from Dr Clare Gerada, chair of the Royal College of General Practitioners, who warned against 'washing dirty linen in public'![78]

In the meantime, there is nothing to stop individual doctors and general practices from choosing to make more information about themselves available to patients. New Zealand general practice has a proud history of innovation – GPs have been early adopters of electronic records and referrals, compared with their peers in other countries.[79] If, as we expect of any other customer-oriented service, a doctor or practice invites patient feedback, audits the quality of services, and operates an effective complaints system, why not make some of that information available on the practice website or in the surgery's waiting room? (General practitioners might also facilitate email communication with patients – a facility that can improve the quality of communication and reduce the need for face-to-face consultations – but that's another story.)[80] Publishing practice information would inform patients and build confidence that a practice is open and committed to quality improvement.

Better checks on doctors

Throughout this book, I have made the claim, backed by survey evidence and my own experience from complaints handling, that patients want to know that doctors are keeping up to date, and that their performance is subject to regular review. The proposed new system for doing this in the United Kingdom has been subject to prolonged and intensive consultation by the General Medical Council, professional and academic debate, and scrutiny from inquiry bodies, notably Dame Janet Smith during the Shipman Inquiry and the House of Commons Health Committee in 2011. Yet in late 2011, more than twelve years after the GMC's commitment to introduce revalidation, the details are still being sorted out, with implementation not scheduled until late 2012.

In the meantime, cases of poorly performing doctors continue to be highlighted in the British media. In October 2011, the BBC Channel 4 *Dispatches* programme asked 'Can you trust your doctor?' and claimed that 'failing doctors routinely slip through the system'.[81] The programme showed film taken secretly in GP practices, where unsuspecting doctors were given case scenarios with classic red flag symptoms that most doctors would easily recognise, but failed to make the correct diagnosis.

Some question the ethics of covert filming of this nature. But Aneez Esmail, the former medical advisor to the Shipman Inquiry who assisted *Dispatches* in preparing the mock case scenarios, justified the secret filming on the basis of the 'overriding public interest'. He claimed that the film revealed 'poor and dangerous practice that the public were totally unaware about, that the quality of general practice was variable, and, frankly, very poor in some areas', and that 'the monitoring of GPs who had been brought before the GMC and who were criticised for poor performance was grossly inadequate'.[82]

I suspect that a similar exercise in New Zealand, targeting doctors who have been subject to multiple complaints, would reveal similarly disturbing results. In 2010, the media highlighted the case of Dr Ratilal Ranchhod, an Auckland medical practitioner working in the community, running a company called 'Housecall' to provide home visits to patients in rest homes and prisons. Dr Ranchhod was well known to the Health and Disability Commissioner, having been the subject of sixteen complaints, making him a very significant outlier. As Commissioner, I had notified the Medical Council three times of my escalating concerns. On the third occasion, I had noted my 'grave concerns that the public is at risk of harm by Dr Ranchhod's ongoing practice' and called for his interim suspension.[83]

When a health ombudsman documents concerns in this way to a medical regulator, it is the equivalent of shouting from the rooftop. Prompted by HDC to undertake a competence review, the Medical Council found that Dr Ranchhod's history taking and examination was brief and cursory, he had 'poorly developed communication skills with a lack of engagement, rapport building, warmth, empathy and compassion', and he was not performing at an acceptable level for a doctor working within a general scope of practice. Yet Dr Ranchhod was allowed to continue practising, subject to strict conditions. The Council admitted that its processes 'take a long time' and justified its decision not to suspend the doctor out of the need to ensure 'fairness to the doctor' and act in a way 'proportionate and appropriate in terms of the doctor'.[84] No wonder that the *Dominion Post* headlined its editorial 'Medical Council failed in its primary role' – of ensuring that medical practitioners are fit to practise.[85]

So, the problems that have led to calls for more rigorous recertification (and for more effective responses by regulators when concerns are raised) persist, especially in cases of isolated doctors working in general practice in the community. As noted, there has been a high level of public scrutiny of revalidation proposals in the United Kingdom. In other countries, the mode of recertification of doctors has been left to medical boards and professional colleges to devise. Some methods are fairly well accepted (notably in Canada) and have good evidence of effectiveness (for example, the maintenance of competence tools developed by the American Board of Internal Medicine). Many useful lessons can be drawn from their experience.

I do not intend to delve into the finer details of optimal recertification regimes.[86] That is an area best left to experts. When cars are subject to a warrant of fitness check in New Zealand or an MOT test in the United Kingdom, our main concern is that only roadworthy cars are passed. We are not concerned to know the precise requirements about brakes and tyres. We have a high degree of confidence, often from personal experience, that if a car is not safe to be on the road, it will fail unless any necessary work is done. In the language of medical appraisal, a warrant of fitness test is 'summative' not 'formative' – we are not simply interested in learning how to improve a car's road safety, we expect a pass or fail decision. The garage authorised to undertake the necessary check *warrants* that the car is fit to be driven on the roads.

I suspect medical readers will be quick to remind me that doctors are not cars and should not be compared to consumer goods – though I well recall the general practitioner who introduced me at a medical association dinner saying, 'Doctors are like cars and sometimes we go through a red light.'[87] (His comments clearly reflected his own recent experience of my investigation, finding shortcomings in his care of a patient.) Doctors are undoubtedly more complex and self-directed than motor vehicles. But if we stay with the roadworthiness analogy for a moment, we want to be reassured that only those doctors who are 'good enough' to remain in practice are recertified – and that for doctors found in need of some upskilling, this will be a condition of their return to practice. We expect the medical regulator to *warrant* their continued fitness to practise.

In the following section, I discuss what recertification currently means in New Zealand and Australia – what steps doctors take to keep up to date, and what checks of ongoing competence medical boards undertake when renewing annual practising certificates. The main message is that the current system largely relies on doctors' self-motivation in undertaking continuing professional development (CPD) activities; that the activities (attending medical update conferences, participating in peer review and audit, and other 'reflective learning') are useful for quality improvement purposes, but do not provide a reliable objective assessment of a doctor's competence; and that any checks undertaken are limited to seeking evidence that claimed activities occurred.

What happens now to recertify doctors?

The law is clear: medical boards are required to check doctors' ongoing competence. Under New Zealand's Health Practitioners Competence Assurance Act 2003, a 'responsible authority' (i.e., a professional regulator, such as the Medical Council) may not register a health practitioner unless satisfied that he or she is 'competent to practise' within their specified scope of practice, nor issue an annual practising certificate 'unless it is satisfied that the applicant meets the required standard of competence'.[88]

In practice, regulators exercise significant discretion in deciding what counts as satisfactory evidence of competence, and use completion of a quota of CPD activities as a proxy for competence. The Medical Council asks applicants for renewal of an annual practising certificate to declare whether they have undertaken 50 hours of CPD in the previous year (including a minimum of 20 hours' CME (continuing medical education) and 10 hours' peer review, and at least one clinical audit) or have fulfilled the requirements of an approved college CPD programme. Ten per cent of self-declarations are audited each year, by requesting further details of the claimed activities.

Responsible authorities in New Zealand are empowered to approve a recertification programme as a mechanism for 'protecting the public from health practitioners who practise below the required standard of competence'[89] and 'ensuring that health practitioners are competent to practise'.[90] A recertification programme may require all or any of the following: passing an exam; completing practical training or a course of instruction; undergoing a review by a designated practitioner of 'clinical and other practices', 'relations with other health practitioners', and clinical records; undergoing an inspection; and undertaking 'a systematic process for ensuring that [the practitioner's services] meet the required standard of competence'.[91] If approved recertification programmes covered all these bases, they might give some surety of competence. In practice, most approved recertification programmes are notably light on exams, review and inspection.

The Australian legislation for health practitioner registration is broadly similar, though with a less pronounced emphasis on competence. A national health practitioner board may register only 'suitably qualified and competent persons' and an applicant for renewal of registration must declare that he or she has 'completed the continuing professional development the applicant was required by an approved registration standard to undertake during the ... preceding period of registration'.[92]

The Medical Board of Australia's *Continuing professional development registration standard* requires doctors to participate regularly in CPD that is 'relevant to their scope of practice in order to maintain, develop, update and enhance their knowledge, skills and performance to ensure that they deliver appropriate and safe care'. CPD must include 'a range of activities to meet individual learning needs including practice-based reflective elements, such as clinical audit, peer-review or performance appraisal, as well as participation in activities to enhance knowledge such as courses, conferences and online learning'.[93]

How do these Australasian recertification requirements translate into practice? As noted, in both countries the regulators mandate CPD. The most common way for a doctor to fulfil his or her CPD requirement is to enrol in a specialty college programme, which helps the practitioner organise and record CPD activity. (Some colleges are beginning to make participation in their own CPD programme mandatory for all Fellows in active practice.) The New Zealand Medical Council has approved the various CPD, CME or MOPS (maintenance of professional standards) programmes run by specialty colleges as approved 'recertification programmes' that satisfy requirements for renewal of a doctor's annual practising certificate. The Medical Board of Australia accepts a doctor's confirmation of having completed an accredited CPD programme within the previous twelve months as satisfactory evidence that the doctor remains competent.

The relevant Australian accreditation standard states that a CPD programme is based on 'self-directed learning' to 'assist participants to maintain and develop knowledge, skills and attitudes essential for meeting the changing needs of patients and the health care delivery system, and for responding to scientific developments in medicine as well as changing societal expectations'.[94] These worthy sentiments are indicative of the level of generality involved in these programmes. They are not like sitting qualification exams.

One example of an approved CPD programme is the MyCPD programme administered by the Royal Australasian College of Physicians.[95] The programme is designed 'to assist participants to keep professionally up-to-date, whilst encouraging participants to plan, record and reflect on professional development needs, as part of their pursuit for lifelong learning'.[96] MyCPD is not an educational resource, but essentially an online repository for recording self-directed learning and reflections. It relies on participants identifying their own professional development needs, planning appropriate activities to meet their needs, and periodically logging into their own MyCPD portfolio to update and record CPD activity.

The majority of doctors who participate in programmes like MyCPD are diligent in undertaking and recording professional activities undertaken to keep up to date. As professionals, they are committed to maintaining their skills. However, medical education experts recognise the limitations of traditional CPD. It measures *activities*, not continued competence. There are many forms of continuing medical education, of varying effectiveness. Contributory factors to effective CPD are said to include active modes of learning (such as doing online modules where learning can be tested), integration of knowledge with everyday practice, and linking CPD to a learning needs analysis.[97]

But this is not how most doctors currently do their CPD. Instead, they tend to rely on 'passive' learning – reading journal articles and online alerts, going to evening lectures and update seminars (sometimes sponsored by pharmaceutical companies), and attending conferences and weekend meetings. Busy doctors schedule these activities at the end of long work days or weeks, and many admit that their concentration and retention is inhibited by tiredness. Even for the most highly motivated doctors, who are not simply totting up the requisite CPD points, keeping up to date is challenging. Teaching sessions and journals help, but modern doctors suffer from information overload and struggle to cope with the stream of the latest guidelines and newly approved medicines.

Another key CPD activity is participation in a peer review group. As noted above, the New Zealand Medical Council requires doctors to undertake ten hours of peer review per year as part of their CPD. Peer review is defined as 'evaluation of the performance of individuals or groups of doctors by members of the same profession or team'.[98] There is clearly educational value for doctors in being able to meet in small groups, in a relatively informal and 'safe' environment, to discuss difficult cases or present reviews of recent journal articles. Peer groups enable participants to reflect on their own practice and to get a sense, from discussion with colleagues, of where they sit in a range of variability. They also provide support, which is especially valuable for practitioners who work in isolation in day-to-day practice. Some peer groups improve doctors' skills in handling difficult situations and help prevent burnout.[99] Thus, peer review can serve both educational and pastoral functions.

However, like other CPD activities, how much a doctor learns from peer review, and how that translates into their practice, depends on their individual professionalism and commitment. A passive participant still earns the requisite CPD points for recertification. Peer review can be relatively unstructured, heavy on discussion and light on evaluation. Sometimes a few controlling members dominate a peer group, and groups may become a forum of discussion of business and social problems rather than learning needs.[100]

The other mandatory part of CPD for doctors in New Zealand is undertaking one clinical audit. This is defined as 'a process used to assess, evaluate and improve the care of patients in a systematic way to enhance health by objectively measuring ... performance against standards'.[101] As with other CPD activities, an audit can be as rigorous or loose as a doctor wishes to make it. In hospital settings, clinical audit is usually organised in a systematic way and involves comparing one's own results over time, and with peers. In community practice, audit may be as basic as a doctor's reviewing a sample of patient records to see whether they meet documentation standards.

Participation in high-quality clinical audit has been identified as a valuable way for doctors to learn and improve their practice, but as currently undertaken by many practitioners it is probably not particularly effective. Experts suggest that, to be useful for recertification purposes, doctors need to participate in well-planned, high-quality, local clinical audit related to their specialty, reflect on the results that relate to their practice, and take action in response to the results.[102] A lot of clinical audit does not meet this standard.[103]

CME, peer review and audit are the main components of CPD for most doctors in New Zealand and Australia. Research confirms what common sense suggests: despite good intentions, many CPD activities are of limited utility in improving practice and targeting areas of suboptimal performance in a doctor's practice, and they don't actually test anything.[104] Conference attendance, local events and journal reading tend to be of greatest value for doctors seeking to keep up to date. One can see that these are valuable activities, to which many doctors devote time and energy. A motivated doctor will learn and adapt their practice, but without an exam or some form of direct observation to assess performance, there is no verification that CPD activity has translated into good practice.

Ian St George spoke for many New Zealand general practitioners when he commented: 'Why do so many of us have a sneaking feeling we are barking up the wrong tree with these recertification activities, participating for the sake of appearances rather than really for the sake of self-improvement?'[105] As St George notes, college CPD programmes were developed to bolster collegiality and transfer the industry concept of continuous quality improvement to medicine. They were not 'set up to *ensure competence* [and] can never *ensure* that [doctors] are competent'.[106]

Before looking at the sort of initiatives under way in other countries to test doctors' competence, one further important factor merits discussion: the difference between a vocationally registered doctor and a general registrant, a doctor registered in a general scope of practice.

The problem of general registrants

For members of the public, a doctor is a doctor. Kay Shirkey, a woman in her forties who attended a local medical centre and saw five different doctors over nine months, before her rare and serious shoulder condition was diagnosed, certainly didn't appreciate that they were general registrants, not vocationally registered general practitioners.[107] Mark Burton, the troubled young mental health consumer who, on discharge from Southland Hospital, promptly killed his mother, probably didn't know that the hospital doctor who cared for him during his six-week admission in the mental health unit was a medical officer working as a psychiatrist, but was not vocationally registered in psychiatry.[108] The Burton family, who had warned the mental health service their son was dangerous, had no idea of the registration status of his main doctor.

Regulatory authorities, in particular the Medical Council and the Health and Disability Commissioner, know that not all doctors are the same. Non-vocationally registered doctors are more likely to be subject to complaints and competence concerns, particularly in general practice.[109] This is hardly surprising, since one would expect the attainment of a specialist qualification and admission as a Fellow of a college to signify a higher level of skills and knowledge. Vocational registration means that a doctor is qualified and permitted to work in a specialist scope of practice.

In hospital settings, good supervision of general registrants can mitigate potential difficulties, although casual locum doctors or medical officers working at specialist level can create problems. Non-vocationally registered medical officers usually work in team settings where they are not isolated, and deficiencies can be detected by colleagues and followed up by the employer requiring remedial actions. Credentialling processes for medical staff working in hospital, although not uniform or consistently applied, are not currently counted for recertification purposes, but anecdotal evidence suggests that they can effectively detect practitioners who are developing competence problems.[110]

However, general registrants working in the community, particularly in solo practices or alongside other non-vocationally trained doctors, may perform poorly without detection. New Zealand, while at the forefront of promoting primary care, lags behind other countries by tolerating general registrants working in general practice. It is unsatisfactory that around one quarter of doctors working in general practice are not vocationally registered, nor working towards vocational registration by participating in a training programme. In Kay Shirkey's case, I commented:

> One has to ask, 'Is this as good as it gets?' In my view, if this is the face of modern primary medical care in New Zealand, it is not a pretty picture. It suggests that for all the fine rhetoric about quality of care, and the emphasis on accreditation of systems, more work is needed to translate that into good care in practice for patients.[111]

The requirement that a general registrant be in a 'collegial relationship' with a vocationally registered doctor who works in a similar type of practice is insufficient to ensure an appropriate standard of patient care, as the Medical Council admits. It is 'too loose and provides no reassurance CPD is occurring'[112] – and in any event, as noted above, CPD on its own provides little reassurance of competence. In the words of former Council chair John Campbell, the current arrangements are 'not a state which can now be justified'.[113] For good reason, the Medical Council is in the process of introducing a new system of 'regular practice review', to be completed every three years for general registrants who are not participating in a vocational training programme.[114]

Regular practice review will require submission of a portfolio of information by the doctor (with details of CPD, audit outcomes and logbooks) and must include some external assessment by peers; it may also include direct observation of consultations, case-based oral assessment, records review, multisource feedback (from peers, patients and colleagues), and interviews with the doctor and colleagues.[115] This is targeted, in-depth assessment of how an 'at risk' doctor actually performs in their day-to-day practice. It is a model of evidence-based assessment of a doctor's fitness for continued practice.

Better models for testing competence

What have countries that have already grappled with these problems done to enact more rigorous recertification and provide greater reassurance to the public? Policy-makers in this area invariably point to the efforts of the Canadian provincial regulators in Quebec, Ontario and Alberta, and the work of a specialty body in the United States, the American Board of Internal Medicine. The North American initiatives are generally more proactive and rigorous than traditional Anglo-Australasian regulatory approaches, which continue to be more focused on reacting to problem doctors than assuring the competence of all doctors.

The power to regulate doctors in Canada is reserved to provincial colleges of physicians and surgeons. Their umbrella body, the Federation of Medical Regulatory Authorities of Canada, has adopted a position statement that 'all licensed physicians in Canada must participate in a recognized revalidation process in which they demonstrate their commitment to continued competent performance in a framework that is fair, relevant, inclusive, transferable and formative'. The wording is revealing. Revalidation is a 'formative' not summative process, which suggests that no one will fail; the definition is hedged about with process qualifications; and it is the 'commitment', rather than the actual performance, that must be demonstrated.

Given the qualified support for revalidation in the statement from the umbrella Federation, I was not entirely surprised to be told by one provincial college registrar: 'Revalidation is a terrible word that has no traction in Canada!'[116] In the face of opposition from medical associations described as 'feral',[117] Canadian provincial regulators have emphasised the need for any system for reviewing physician competence to be professionally supported and to have a quality improvement focus. This emphasis is nicely captured in the name of the Alberta PAR programme. The 'A' between the 'P' for Physician and the 'R' for Review stands for Achievement, not Assessment or Assurance, as I had assumed.

That said, the Canadians have invested significant resources in developing sophisticated tools for reviewing physician competence, and the gradual acceptance of their use by the profession suggests that an incremental approach has much to commend it. The assessment processes complement mandatory CPD that most doctors complete via the two national certifying bodies for family physicians and other specialists.[118] Regulators have developed a pyramid model of 'Maintenance and Enhancement of Physician Performance',[119] although it has been implemented in different ways. The underlying rationale is well described by Norman and colleagues:

> Using an epidemiologic analogy, it could be argued that the 'disease' of incompetence has such a low prevalence that no single testing method is likely to be cost-effective. Instead, a relicensure process shows promise if it contains multiple components: first, a relatively economical screening phase with high sensitivity (but possibly low specificity), then a diagnostic phase ... and finally a treatment phase ...[120]

In Quebec, the provincial regulator, the Collège des Médecins du Québec, fortified by research indicating that 94 per cent of a randomly selected group of 100 family physicians were providing good-to-excellent quality care,[121] decided to target its stage one screening efforts on 'at risk' doctors. They include doctors still practising more than 35 years since obtaining their medical degree; doctors who are significant outliers based on their prescribing and billing data (to which the Quebec College, uniquely amongst regulators, has access); specialists doing only office-based work and no hospital work; international medical graduates with restricted permits; and doctors subject to complaints and concerns. This approach is consistent with evidence that increasing years in practice is associated with diminished performance,[122] and attuned to other red flags for potential problems.

The targeted doctors in Quebec receive a 'professional inspection visit' that involves review by a peer physician inspector of a sample of the doctor's clinical records and a visit (possibly with direct observation of consultations), leading to a written report with feedback and recommendations. In the minority of cases where serious concerns are identified, the doctor may be required to undertake an intensive remedial programme and be subject to practice restrictions in the meantime. The Quebec system is much lauded by other medical regulators (who envy the College's access to utilisation data), and represents a pragmatic (and less resource-intensive) response to quality assurance of the medical profession, but it does not attempt to ensure that every doctor in Quebec with a practice permit is practising safely.

The College of Physicians and Surgeons of Ontario has implemented a peer assessment programme for all doctors. Since 1980, thousands of doctors in Ontario have had their skills assessed by a fellow doctor. This involves a practice visit by a peer assessor, who reviews patient records and has a discussion with the doctor (e.g., about the management of a case from the reviewed records). A formal assessment report follows.

With a population of 25,000 practising doctors, it has not yet been practicable for the College to peer assess all doctors. Currently, all doctors upon turning 70 (and thereafter every five years), and a random sample of doctors on the register, undergo a peer assessment. In 2010, there were 1625 peer assessments performed on doctors in Ontario; 66 per cent of these were a random selection from the register.[123] The aim, from 2015, is to have every doctor assessed every ten years.[124]

Post-assessment surveys indicate that more than 80 per cent of assessed Ontario doctors find the process is educational and adds value. If problems are identified, a more intensive review is undertaken, including an interview with a College committee, and possibly a further assessment with observations of actual consultations or procedures. In rare cases (fewer than ten per year) where, during assessment, a doctor refuses to co-operate or there is evidence of incompetence or a risk of patient safety, the doctor is referred to an investigations committee indicating a concern. The information gathered during the assessment is privileged by statute and can not be disclosed to the investigations committee. The Ontario College believes its processes detect most clinical performance problems, but they are not designed to pick up communication deficits (other than written communication deficits apparent in patient records). The assessment system that best detects these sorts of problem is Alberta's.

The College of Physicians & Surgeons of Alberta requires every practising doctor to undergo a Performance Achievement Review (PAR) every five years.[125] The novel feature of PAR in Alberta (now adopted in Nova Scotia on a seven-year cycle, and pending in Manitoba) is that the assessment is based on multisource feedback (sometimes called 360-degree feedback). In the case of a family physician, feedback is sought from 25 patients, eight co-workers, and eight medical colleagues (selected by the doctor), together with the doctor's self-appraisal. The questions relate primarily to the doctor's communication skills, co-ordination of care and collegiality, although medical colleagues are also asked to assess clinical competence. The results are analysed by an independent company and the doctor receives a written report showing their mean (on a 1 to 5 scale) for the various indicators and how they compare with other doctors.

Under Alberta's PAR programme, 20 per cent of doctors (the top 5%, the bottom 10%, and another 5% where the doctor indicates difficulties with stress) are followed up with telephone interviews, and a small number (around 3% to 4% of the total group) progress to a practice visit. If there are serious concerns, the doctor is required to undergo a more intensive assessment. The entire process has a strong quality improvement focus and is kept separate from the College's complaints and disciplinary processes. PAR is also separate from the peer review/practice visit process for doctors where the College has been alerted to clinical competence concerns.

Critics point out that PAR is 'designed to foster quality improvement, but it lacks an external standard for "passing"'.[126] Clearly, it does not purport to test competence, but common sense suggests that if a doctor receives poor ratings from medical colleagues for competence, from co-workers for collegiality, or from patients for communication skills, further scrutiny is warranted to see if the doctor has some performance problems. Yet when an adaptation of PAR was trialled in New Zealand in 2007, in a poorly designed Pilot Performance Evaluation Programme, it was rejected after medical critics claimed the pilot seemed to show 'patients are not particularly good at knowing whether a doctor is a good doctor'.[127] At a time in health care when all the rhetoric is about 'patient voice' and 'patient-centred care', it defies belief that tentative steps to include patient input in multisource feedback on doctors' skills should be rejected because 'Patients fail in doctor diagnosis', as the New Zealand experiment was headlined in the media.[128]

Canada offers some interesting possibilities for recertification of doctors. But there is force to the rhetorical question posed by Wendy Levinson, 'Revalidation of physicians in Canada: Are we passing the test?' Levinson concludes that 'to assure our colleagues and the public', revalidation should include 'an external assessment of physician competence', with a secure exam (to assess knowledge) and a practice review with input from peers and patients (to assess actual performance).[129] However, any suggestion of exams for recertification is anathema to the medical profession in Canada.[130] Canadian regulators continue to search for the 'Holy Grail' of 'valid methodology to measure the actual performance of physicians in practice'.[131]

Maintenance of certification in the United States

Experts in the United States are well advanced in finding the Holy Grail of effective performance assessment of practising physicians. The Federation of State Medical Boards has adopted a Maintenance of Licensure framework, making it a condition of licence renewal that physicians 'should provide evidence of participation in a program of professional development and lifelong learning',[132] but it has been left to medical specialty boards to put the flesh on the bones of these requirements. More than 85 per cent of practising physicians in the United States are board-certified specialists,[133] since hospitals and payers usually require board certification. Specialty boards require regular renewal of certification (between six and ten years) and have developed sophisticated tools for Maintenance of Certification (MOC).

The umbrella American Board of Medical Specialties (with 24 member boards) requires MOC programmes to incorporate four components: evidence of good professional standing through an unrestricted licence and multisource feedback from patients and peers; participation in lifelong learning (self-assessment modules); passing a secure examination of cognitive and clinical problem-solving skills; and assessment of practice performance.[134] Eric Holmboe and colleagues at the American Board of Internal Medicine (ABIM, the largest specialty board in the United States, covering more than one quarter of all physicians) have undertaken the leading work on maintenance of competence.

The ABIM work is underpinned by good evidence that practitioner skills decay with time,[135] physicians' ability to assess their own skills is poor,[136] and less than 30 per cent of physicians examine their performance data and try to improve on their own.[137] Hence the ABIM MOC programme includes two critical elements: an actual exam, which focuses on clinical problem-solving and diagnosis based on cases relevant to the doctor's clinical practice; and Practice Improvement Modules (PIMs) that require doctors to conduct an audit of some aspect of their practice, collect patient feedback, and assess their practice system. Data is submitted to ABIM for analysis, feedback is provided (comparing the doctor's performance with guidelines), an improvement plan is implemented, and performance is then re-measured to check for improvement. Physicians often experience a valuable 'aha!' moment when receiving PIM feedback that reveals an unexpected gap in their performance.[138]

The ABIM approach faces vigorous opposition from many internists critical of its relevance and the time and expense involved.[139] No doubt it will continue to be refined. But the MOC model can be justified on the grounds of accountability to the public (who look to board certification as evidence of competence)[140] and quality improvement (since there is a growing body of research evidence showing a positive association between maintenance of certification and quality of care).[141] Holmboe argues persuasively that 'a multifaceted physician-level performance assessment system has substantial potential to align the public's need and desire to ensure their physician is competent, at the minimum, with providing the physician with meaningful, actionable information and data to improve performance'.[142]

Revalidation in the United Kingdom

No medical regulator in the world has prepared for revalidation as assiduously as the General Medical Council in the United Kingdom. Revalidation is defined in the Medical Act 1983 (UK) as an 'evaluation of a medical practitioner's fitness to practise'.[143] The GMC describes revalidation as a process to assure patients and the public, employers and other healthcare practitioners that licensed doctors are up to date and practising to the appropriate professional standards. Doctors who are unable to demonstrate this will lose their licence to practise.

Revalidation has been on the agenda for twelve years in the UK, after a substantial majority of the GMC agreed, in February 1999, to its introduction. Why has something seemingly so simple proved so complicated? The delays have resulted from lack of clarity about the purpose of revalidation; disagreement over its form and content; vigorous opposition from within the profession to the imposition of perceived bureaucratic, external controls; and cost concerns.

Implementation of a modest form of revalidation was pending in 2004, when Dame Janet Smith, in her Shipman Inquiry report,[144] damned the GMC's proposals as inadequate to give the public real reassurance of a licensed doctor's fitness to practise. This in turn led to Chief Medical Officer Liam Donaldson's 2006 report *Good Doctors, Safer Patients*[145] and the Government's 2007 White Paper *Trust, Assurance and Safety – The Regulation of Health Professionals in the 21st Century*,[146] which have shaped the current proposals.

The GMC is now well advanced in its plans, with pilots being trialled. During a major consultation in 2010, five key themes emerged: revalidation needs to be 'as streamlined, straightforward and proportionate as possible'; the model must be flexible; costs must be minimised (a major concern given cost pressures on the NHS); further detail is needed before revalidation is rolled out; and the proposed models need further testing and evaluation.

One of the first actions of the new coalition government Health Secretary, Andrew Lansley, in May 2010 was to ask the GMC to delay revalidation, so that the pilots could be extended – while expressing support for its introduction. In October 2010, the GMC and all four Departments of Health issued a Statement of Intent, committing to launch revalidation across the United Kingdom in late 2012. The House of Commons Health Committee in early 2011 called for 'no further delays', stated that 'the primary purpose of revalidation is to protect the interests of patients' (thus remediation of problem doctors can be only a secondary concern), and recommended that appraisal processes be streamlined and integrated into existing appraisal and clinical governance systems operated by employers.[147]

The plan is that every licensed doctor in the United Kingdom will be required to be revalidated every five years. A local 'responsible officer' will make a recommendation to the GMC about whether a doctor should be revalidated. The recommendation will be based on the results of the doctor's annual appraisals. These, in turn, will be based on the doctor's CPD portfolio, supplemented by multisource feedback from patients and colleagues. If the GMC is not satisfied that a doctor should be revalidated, he or she will be subject to 'fitness to practise' processes (in the same way as a doctor who is subject to a serious complaint or competence concerns), which may result in loss of their licence to practise.

In December 2010, I joined leading experts from the United Kingdom, the Netherlands, the United States, Canada and New Zealand in London at an international symposium entitled 'Revalidation: Contributing to the evidence base'. The meeting provided valuable insights into the slow progress towards mandatory revalidation of doctors in the United Kingdom – and lessons for medical regulators in other countries.

Despite the general support for revalidation, there was a lack of agreement as to its purpose. The most commonly expressed concern remains that revalidation will be used to weed out 'bad apples' and that it is not sensitive enough to do that effectively. Most participants agreed that the primary purpose is to give the public assurance that a licensed doctor meets minimum standards, and is thus 'good enough'; but that a second, not inconsistent, purpose is to improve the quality of medical practice overall.

A recurrent theme was the need to make a start, accepting that the tools used in revalidation will become more robust over time. Participation in CPD and clinical audit will certainly form part of appraisal and revalidation processes. There is a lot of nervousness about the use of multisource feedback, especially feedback from patients (one leading doctor commented, 'I don't want to be rated if it means I can't tell you to stop eating buns!'), but the consensus is that a number of questionnaires are sufficiently robust to be used for revalidation. Patient feedback is an important 'report on experience', and colleague feedback provides reliable information about a doctor's performance.[148] However, care is needed in the interpretation and use of multisource feedback, given the risk of systematic bias related to the characteristics of the assessors giving feedback and the personal characteristics of the doctor being assessed.[149]

I came away from the London symposium convinced that revalidation of doctors will become a reality in the United Kingdom over the next couple of years; that international experience suggests it takes at least a decade to introduce such a major change; that how reforms are communicated to the medical profession is critical, given the cultural shift involved; and that regulators face enormous pressure to water down reforms to be palatable to the profession.

My recertification prescription

What lessons can New Zealand and Australia learn from revalidation and maintenance of competence reforms in North America and the United Kingdom? Both Antipodean countries are well placed to implement effective recertification of doctors. Legislation imposes clear duties on health practitioner boards to ensure that health practitioners remain competent before renewing their practising certificate. The title of New Zealand's Health Practitioners Competence Assurance Act sends the clearest possible signal of what the public has the right to expect.

I have argued that the current practice of the New Zealand Medical Council and the Medical Board of Australia does not give the public adequate assurance that every licensed doctor is competent. Both regulators rely too heavily on self-assessed CPD activities as sufficient evidence that a doctor is practising safely. Their proactive efforts to check on competence are weak. Even when reacting to notified concerns, their response is sometimes slow and relatively ineffective, overly risk-averse, and more concerned with the doctor's legal rights and remediation than patient safety.

What changes do I recommend to enhance recertification?

1. Regulators must be clear about their role. They must send a very clear signal that they take their public protective function seriously, and that the primary purpose of recertification is to ensure that every licensed doctor remains competent and fit to practise. Yes, this should be done in a way that supports doctors' own professionalism and within a quality improvement framework, but the minimum standards of *Good Medical Practice* endorsed by regulators[150] must be enforced. Remediation of doctors, though an important aim, should not obscure the overriding goal of protecting the public by ensuring proper standards in the practice of medicine.

2. Recertification based on the current Australasian models of CPD is inadequate. The choice of CPD as a marker for competent practice may be defensible on grounds of pragmatism and expense, but it does not absolve boards of their duty to ensure that every licensed practitioner remains fully competent. The New Zealand Medical Council acknowledges the need to improve in this area; its first strategic goal is to '[o]ptimise mechanisms to ensure that doctors are competent and fit to practise'.[151]

If medical boards continue to rely on approved college CPD programmes as evidence of ongoing competence, they must use their regulatory levers to prompt colleges and professional societies to modernise their CPD programmes so they incorporate some of the best features of the emerging North American and United Kingdom models. The New Zealand Council has called for doctors' professional organisations to 'step up' their monitoring of doctors' performance to retain public confidence.[152] Work undertaken by the Royal Australasian College of Surgeons to develop a *Surgical Competence and Performance* guide[153] is promising, as is a similar project by the Royal Australasian College of Physicians, with patterns of behavioural markers ('good' and 'poor') identified for nine key competencies, but it is still too generic and formative to give a reliable assessment of a doctor's performance in clinical practice.

Regulators also need to further specify the requirements for CPD, articulating minimum standards for continuing medical education, clinical audit and peer review. The specifications should be based on the expertise of colleges in developing components that are educationally valid and will help doctors improve their work, without being onerous and burdensome. New regulatory initiatives will succeed only if supported by the profession. Thus, professional bodies must be asked to develop evidence-based processes to assess performance, in ways doctors will find relevant and worthwhile – a better use of their time than current methods. The new processes should supplant (and not be additional to) current methods.

For doctors working in public hospitals, recertification should build on, and not duplicate, checks that already occur as part of credentialling processes and clinical governance systems. However, until credentialling and clinical governance become more consistent and rigorous than at present, they cannot be relied on as assurance that all medical staff in hospitals are practising at an acceptable standard.

At some point in the future, Anglo-Canadian-Australasian doctors will need to overcome their aversion to periodic exams, given the evidence that they clearly add value in testing cognitive and clinical problem-solving skills. It makes no sense that in all countries passing exams is required for a medical degree and specialist qualification, yet only in the United States is it considered a mandatory component of recertification as a specialist. At the moment, it is a bridge too far, but over time the value of exams will inevitably lead to their incorporation as one part of recertification.

In the meantime, multisource feedback from patients, co-workers and colleagues must be included as a component of CPD for recertification purposes. Patients want to be able to give feedback about their doctors,[154] in particular about their communication skills, and they expect to have a voice in recertification processes.[155] Good doctors will want to hear what their patients, co-workers and colleagues say about them, provided that the information is fed back in a constructive and meaningful way.

3. Unless medical regulators propose to undertake periodic performance assessment of all doctors, as is planned in Ontario and is pending (via the appraisal system) in the United Kingdom, they need to implement targeted screening of 'at risk' doctors along the

lines adopted in Quebec. The New Zealand Medical Council's planned regular practice review processes for general registrants (who are not in a vocational training programme)[156] is a promising move in this direction, and needs to be implemented in a rigorous way.[157] The Council should consider requiring a regular practice review (rather than simply relying on CPD compliance) for other doctors such as those who, by virtue of years in practice or red flags of complaints or concerns, merit closer scrutiny because they may pose a risk to patients. Use of these sorts of tools should be promoted vigorously, and the Council should take a bolder stance than has traditionally been evident in its attempts to initiate 'competence reviews'[158] in response to notified concerns.

Reformed regulators to protect the public

Action on my information and recertification prescriptions will go a long way to ensure better information for patients, and provide reassurance that doctors are keeping up to date and meeting patient expectations. Both will help build patients' trust in their own doctor and public confidence in the medical profession. However, more needs to be done to demonstrate to the public that medical regulators are independent of the profession, are transparent and accountable, and are performing their regulatory functions effectively.

In Part 3, I argued that medical regulators are characteristically 'reluctant regulators' whose passive resistance to change has slowed progress towards the goal of assuredly good doctors expected by the public. Boards tend to be conservative, too close to the medical profession they are appointed to regulate, and unduly focused on remediation at the expense of public protection and accountability. They do a passable job at reacting to concerns about poor performance, and have yet to demonstrate rigour in proactively checking doctors' competence.

WHAT CAN WE IMPROVE?

The changes in governance of the General Medical Council, and in the approach now evident in the GMC's work, are illuminating. The GMC states on its website: 'We are not here to protect the medical profession – their interests are protected by others. Our job is to protect patients.'[159] A concerted effort by the reformed GMC to become more visible and more proactive in its work is starting to pay dividends. One sign is that there has been a sharp increase in the number of doctors referred to the GMC by medical directors, patients and public bodies. There is no evidence that doctors' standards in the United Kingdom have dropped; rather, people appear to have increased confidence that reporting a concern will prompt action. A survey of 100 medical directors in the UK cited greater awareness of and commitment to high professional standards, with doctors more willing to report concerns.[160] This is an encouraging sign if it means that performance problems amongst doctors, when they cannot be satisfactorily resolved in the workplace, are being reported rather than remaining hidden behind closed doors. Tolerance for poor performance appears to be waning.

The notable changes to the General Medical Council have been the move to parity of lay and medical members on the governing council; ensuring that all Council members are appointed by an independent appointments commission;[161] and greater accountability by requiring annual reports to Parliament (and oversight by the Health Select Committee of the House of Commons) and a watchdog role over the Council's processes by an independent body, the Council for Healthcare Regulatory Excellence. These changes have dramatically reformed the GMC. From my own observation of its recent work, the GMC is taking a noticeably different tack, with greater openness, a tougher stance on doctors' duties and more of an outward focus. Its first 'state of medicine' report has been well received and shows a modern regulator entering dialogue with the profession, patients, employers and the body politic.[162] It has issued new guidance to doctors on *Raising and acting on concerns about patient safety*.[163] Although it is early days, and there continue to be media reports alleging inadequate responses to fitness to practise concerns,[164] the GMC appears to be building professional and public confidence.

My regulatory reform prescription

What changes can be made to improve the independence, transparency, accountability and effectiveness of medical regulators?[165]

1. The relevant legislation should be amended to require parity of lay and health practitioner members on the governing councils of health practitioner regulators, and appointments should be made through a transparent and independent process, with members appointed for their skills in governance and their ability to contribute to the performance of the public protective functions of a regulator. No places on the board should be reserved for election by the profession. The job of a regulator must be clearly seen to be to regulate the profession in the public interest, not on behalf of the profession.

    These changes will both make regulators more effective in their work, improving corporate governance and bringing a better skill mix to boards, and tackle the public perception that whenever a decision is made that appears to be lenient towards the doctor, it must have resulted from doctors 'looking after their own'. The proposed reforms would be visible evidence of a shift from classic self-regulation to a model of co-regulation or shared regulation,[166] which better serves the public interest.

2. Legislative reform is also needed to make medical regulators subject to freedom of information laws, in the same way that other public sector agencies are. Careful consideration will need to be given to appropriate protection of individual patient and doctor privacy interests. However, subject to this important caveat, there should be

a presumption that it is in the public interest to make information about the outcome of regulators' work publicly available.

This change will ensure greater transparency and help lift the current veil of secrecy over regulatory processes. It needs to be matched by more visible evidence of accountability. Legislation in New Zealand and Australia already requires medical boards to file annual reports with the Minister of Health, and for them to be tabled in Parliament, but the Health Select Committees of Parliament need to take a much more active role in holding boards to account by public hearings and public reports critiquing their work.[167]

Accountability can also be promoted by other means. There may be scope to broaden the functions of established bodies, such as the healthcare complaint commissions in Australia and the Health and Disability Commissioner in New Zealand, to report on the performance of health practitioner regulators. However, this could create problematic tensions in the current co-regulatory arrangements between commissions and regulators. A new watchdog body like the Council for Healthcare Regulatory Excellence (CHRE) in the United Kingdom has much to commend it, although given fiscal pressures on government health spending, it would need to be funded by professional levies. CHRE has withstood bonfires of quangos (quasi-autonomous non-governmental organisations) in the United Kingdom, since it is widely acknowledged that having an independent watchdog over the regulators has improved the quality of their work and engendered greater public confidence in regulatory processes.

3. Health practitioner regulators should be required to work more closely together, to reap the benefits of shared thinking and best practice in professional regulation. Australia is well placed to achieve this objective with its overarching Australian Health

Practitioner Regulation Agency, which supports the work of each of the national health practitioner boards. New Zealand has an excellent framework for common approaches to health practitioner regulation, in the Health Practitioners Competence Assurance Act 2003, but the various boards currently operate quite independently, with differing approaches to key issues such as competence reviews and recertification. Although it is important not to lose professional identity, it would make a great deal of sense for regulators to share expertise and agree on and implement the most effective, evidence-based means of ensuring ongoing competence and fitness to practise across all professions.[168]

Regulation is expensive and time-consuming, and many regulators currently spread limited resources very thinly across their whole profession. A case can be made for more evidence-based regulation, so that regulatory resources (and the burden on practitioners) are focused on areas where they will make the most difference, along the lines of the 'right-touch' regulation promoted by the Council for Healthcare Regulatory Excellence in the UK.[169] Emerging research suggests that it may be possible to identify the 5 per cent group of 'high risk doctors', and focus interventions there, while minimising the regulatory burden on the bulk (95%) of 'good enough' doctors.[170] By combining resources, and adopting more sophisticated, evidence-based regulatory approaches, health practitioner boards can become more effective in protecting the public and guiding their professions.

An effective prescription?

How can I be confident that my prescription for change will improve the current state of affairs: result in better information for patients and the public, justified reassurance that doctors remain competent, and enhanced public trust in the medical profession and its watchdog bodies? What chance do my recommendations stand of being adopted, given the history of professional resistance to external regulation?

First, my proposals are consistent with patient and public expectations, which will inevitably grow louder over time. I believe they reflect what patients want. They are specifically targeted at weaknesses in the present system, which allow substandard doctors to continue in practice. They seek to circumvent the major roadblocks that have delayed necessary change, and to bolster public confidence in doctors and medical watchdogs.

Secondly, my recommendations are practical and achievable – as is evident from the various ways in which they are being accepted internationally. These changes are already happening in parts of North America, and are imminent in the United Kingdom. They can be implemented in a way that is not burdensome, unfair, expensive or time-consuming for ordinary practitioners. Responsive regulators can make the proposals work for patients, doctors, other key players in the health system, and the public.

Finally, my prescription for change is designed to support, not undermine, medical professionalism. There are many intangible elements in the patient–doctor relationship, and not everything of value can be counted and measured. Nor can the profession be expected to jump through hoops simply because external agencies demand proof of trustworthiness and competence. The best reason for changes along the lines I have argued for is to honour the profession's commitment to maintenance of competence. This is an obligation of public service generated by the profession itself. It is in keeping with the trust that most patients continue to invest in their doctor.

EPILOGUE

I opened this book saying that I would try to explain why the simple aim of ensuring that every licensed doctor is a good doctor has proven so difficult to achieve – and to suggest the steps that need to be taken to meet the modest expectations of patients. I end it optimistic that change can be achieved.

Writing the book has helped me clarify my own thinking about good doctors. I gained insights from my research and interviews with experts, but also from numerous conversations about the topic. I sat with my own general practitioner, at the end of his long and busy work day, and quizzed him for over an hour about how he keeps up to date. I put the same question to my doctor friends. They are only too aware that current CPD methods are far from perfect – but are trying their best to cope with a tidal wave of new information and increasing demands from funders and government agencies. I was struck by the fragility of their belief in their own knowledge, skills and expertise. Their professional self-esteem and motivation could easily wilt, and they could simply pack their bags and seek other work, if the wrong sorts of changes are enacted. We would all be the poorer if that happened.

Re-reading some of the cases from my time as Health and Disability Commissioner brought back many memories. Intolerable, unbearable things happen to some patients. They and their families show courage and determination in bringing a complaint, looking for answers and trying to stop the same thing happening to someone else. Often they are victims of a complex chain of events – injured when all the holes in the Swiss cheese line up to allow a trajectory of error. Some patients are let down by incompetent doctors who should not have been allowed to practise, yet were able to do so because colleagues, employers and regulators turned a blind eye or succumbed to pressure not to intervene. Even if no physical harm ensues to patients, why should they receive second-rate care from doctors whose poor standards should never have been tolerated?

It is a gift for patients and families to allow their stories to be told. One case that I related in Part 2 involved Ms A, the loyal patient of the elderly suburban doctor, Dr B, who failed to take the basic steps that should have detected her uterine tumour much earlier. I described it as an 'ordinary failure', but also a private scandal. In making final revisions to my book, I called Ms A's sister to check whether she was happy for the case to be used in this way. It is nine years since Ms A died. But her sister said that, whenever the family gathers, they still talk about what happened. 'It should never have happened. She *trusted* her doctor – she had been going to him for over 20 years.' I thanked the family for being willing to let the story be told. 'Thank *you*,' Ms A's sister said, 'I just hope that things change.'[1]

While writing my book, I have watched friends and family cope with their own medical crises. Time and again, I have been reminded of the qualities that make good doctors. Are they simply writing scripts for the latest wonder medication, without fully engaging the patient in making a decision about whether it's the right course of action? What steps do they (or their practice nurse) take to ensure the patient understands what signs and symptoms to watch out for, and what to do if they eventuate? Where multiple providers are involved, does the primary doctor make sure that the care is properly co-ordinated? At the most basic level, does the doctor listen to the patient, and create the space to allow him or her to reveal private fears and worries?

I was always clear that my book would be entitled 'The Good Doctor', but I played with various subtitles before opting for the simple phrase 'What Patients Want'. Just before the book went to print, I showed the cover to my father, who spends more time with doctors these days than he would wish. 'Yes,' he said, 'what patients want. But it should also say, "and need".' He made a good point. The changes that I have argued for are not fluffy extras to appease noisy patients or earnest policy wonks. They are intended to meet the legitimate needs of patients. And they are fully consistent with the aims of medical professionalism, and the purposes of modern 'right-touch' regulation.[2]

Of course, I know that changing established ways of doing things is not easy. Apparently straightforward policy reforms can mask a world of complications. I like the irony of Glenn Colquhoun, a New Zealand doctor and poet, in this poem:

A brief format to be used when consulting with patients

The patient will talk.

The doctor will talk.

The doctor will listen while
the patient is talking.

The patient will listen while
the doctor is talking.

The patient will think that the doctor
knows what the doctor is talking about.

The doctor will think that the patient
knows what the patient is talking about.

The patient will think that the doctor
knows what the patient is talking about.

> The doctor will think that the patient
> knows what the doctor is talking about.
>
> The doctor will be sure.
> The patient will be sure.
>
> The patient will be sure.
> The doctor will be sure.
>
> Shouldn't hurt a bit, should it?[3]

Justified reassurance for patients may not come easily. A decade of birthing pains in the United Kingdom confirms that making changes to help ensure 'good doctors, safer patients'[4] may hurt a bit. New ways of providing better information for patients and the public, undertaking more effective checks of competence, and ensuring that regulators do their job properly, will be challenging.

I hope that readers of my book will be persuaded by the need for reforms so that our trust in doctors, and our confidence in regulatory systems, is well placed. I look forward to the day when we can all rely on the public medical register and a current licence to practise medicine as assurance that any licensed doctor is competent. We do not want to take 'pot luck'. We want to know that every doctor is 'good enough', a professional in whom we can be sure.

ACKNOWLEDGEMENTS

I have dedicated this book to my friends Mike Taggart and Charlotte Paul. A close friend from law school days, Mike always encouraged my interest in law and medicine. He urged me to 'write the book you want to write', and that is what I've tried to do. Charlotte has taught me much about public health, ethics and human nature over many years, and was my constant companion on this book journey. Her insights into professionalism and the complexities of the patient–doctor relationship have helped shape my thinking.

I am grateful to the New Zealand Law Foundation for the award of an International Research Fellowship, which funded my research and travel in preparing the book, and gave me the luxury of a year's study leave. I thank the Foundation for its support, in particular Lynda Hagen and Dianne Gallagher for their encouragement. I am also grateful to the University of Auckland, and successive Deans of Law, Paul Rishworth and Andrew Stockley, for the grant of research leave to complete the book.

I was fortunate to be a Visiting Scholar at the Nuffield Trust in London and the Hastings Center in New York, while undertaking research in 2010. Marylebone, London and Garrison, New York are lovely locations in which to think, talk and write. Staff from each of these institutions helped me, but I owe special thanks to Judith Smith (Nuffield) and Nancy Berlinger, Dan Callahan and Tom Murray (Hastings). I also enjoyed fruitful research periods at Melbourne University and Otago University.

Staff of the General Medical Council in London, and the Medical Council of New Zealand in Wellington, have been especially helpful. My thanks to Niall Dickson and Una Lane of the GMC for sharing their time and expertise, and allowing me access to the resources and staff of the Council. John Adams, Ian Brown, Joan Crawford and Michael Thorn from the MCNZ were always willing to answer my questions and give me pointers for further research.

I was also fortunate to visit medical colleges in Quebec, Ontario and Alberta. Many staff gave me valuable time, but I owe special thanks to Andre Jacques (Collège des Médecins du Québec), Jerome Frank (Royal College of Physicians and Surgeons of Canada), Rocco Gerace and Dan Faulkner (College of Physicians and Surgeons of Ontario), and Trevor Theman (College of Physicians and Surgeons of Alberta). Closer to home, I was helped by key staff at the Australian Health Practitioner Regulation Agency, including Martin Fletcher, and the chair of the Medical Board of Australia, Joanna Flynn.

I am grateful to many other doctors, patient advocates, health policy-makers and scholars who gave me their time and shared their ideas, including Judith Allsop, Carol Black, Ben Bridgewater, Harry Cayton, Angela Coulter, Liam Donaldson, Joan Higgins, Donald Irvine, Martin Marshall, Alastair Scotland, Anna van der Gaag and Kieran Walshe (in the United Kingdom), and Marie Bismark, Kerry Breen, Ian Freckelton and David Studdert (in Australia).

From a wide cast of contributors in New Zealand, I thank my own doctor, Chris Dominick, my friend Mary Seddon and my academic mentor Peter Skegg. I gratefully acknowledge New Zealand doctor and poet Glenn Colquhoun for permission to quote his poem 'A brief format to be used when consulting with patients'.

Several friends and colleagues commented on drafts of the book. They are not responsible for the shortcomings that remain, but each contributed insights and challenged my claims. They have undoubtedly improved the finished product. Many thanks to Marie Bismark, Joanna Manning, Charlotte Paul, Sara Rishworth, Nicola Sladden and Judi Strid.

Auckland University Press was immediately enthusiastic about my book proposal. I am grateful to publisher Sam Elworthy and editor Anna Hodge for their advice and professionalism. Writer Simon Hertnon helped me sort out the structure of the book and was a source of encouragement along the way. In the final stages, I was ably assisted by Louise Belcher in checking citations, Mike Wagg in copyediting, and Anne Russell in proofreading the text and compiling the index.

Those closest to me have lived with the book, and endured frequent conversations about its progress, over the past eighteen months. I thank Greg and my family, especially my doctor brother Graham and my parents, for being such a great support team.

This book reflects what I have learnt over many years from numerous complaints made by patients and families, brought in the hope that the same thing won't happen to someone else, and from the countless good doctors I have encountered, who strive to provide the competent and compassionate care that patients want and deserve. I thank them all for their inspiration.

Ron Paterson
Kawakawa Bay, January 2012

NOTES

PREFACE

1. I first presented some of the material in this book at a General Medical Council symposium in London in December 2010. See General Medical Council, *Publication of Proceedings. International Revalidation Symposium: Contributing to the evidence base*, London, 2011.
2. Under the New Zealand Code, any person – the 'consumer', a family member or even a third party such as another health practitioner – can complain that a provider of health or disability services failed to comply with the duties (of respect, care and communication, etc.) set out in the 10 rights prescribed under the Code. A complaint may be made to the provider direct, to a consumer advocate, or to the Health and Disability Commissioner (HDC). In the event of a complaint to HDC, the Commissioner has wide powers in dealing with the complaint, including referring the matter to a registration authority ('if it appears from the complaint that the competence of a health practitioner or his or her fitness to practise ... may be in doubt': the Health and Disability Commissioner Act 1994, s. 34(1)(a)) or undertaking a formal investigation. An investigation by the Commissioner may result in a finding that the provider breached the consumer's rights, and may trigger professional discipline or a claim before the Human Rights Review Tribunal. For an overview of the New Zealand Code and the complaints system, see R. Paterson, 'The patients' complaints system in New Zealand', *Health Affairs*, vol. 21, 2002, pp. 70–79.
3. The one-year risk of referral to the National Clinical Assessment Service in England is approximately 0.5% for all doctors and rises to 1% for those in senior posts (L. Donaldson, *Good Doctors, Safer Patients: Proposals to strengthen the system to assure and improve the performance of doctors and to protect the safety of patients. A report by the Chief Medical Officer*, Department of Health: London, 2006). Marilynn Rosenthal estimates that between 3% and 5% of practising doctors are incompetent, based on her qualitative research on doctors in the United Kingdom and Sweden in 1990 (M. Rosenthal, *The Incompetent Doctor: Behind closed doors*, Open University Press: Buckingham, 1995). In the United States, Leape and Fromson estimate that '[w]hen all conditions are considered, *at least one third of all physicians will experience, at some time in their career, a period during which they have a condition that impairs their ability to practice medicine safely*; for a hospital with a staff of 100 physicians, this translates to an average of 1 to 2 physicians per year' (L. Leape and J. Fromson, 'Problem doctors: Is there a system-level solution?', *Annals of Internal Medicine*, vol. 144, 2006, pp. 107–15 at p. 109 [emphasis in original]). Researchers in Ontario, Canada, testing competence assessment tools, estimate that 15 out of 1000 (1.5%) randomly selected physicians will be found to have very serious problems that require mandatory education, and 5 out of 1000 (0.5%) will require removal from practice (G. Norman et al., 'Competency assessment of primary care physicians as part of a peer review program', *Journal of the American Medical Association*, vol. 270, 1993, pp. 1046–51).

NOTES TO PAGES X-4

4   A. J. Cronin, *The Citadel*, The New English Library: London, 1965, p. 160.
5   I note that since July 2010 I have served as a community board member of the Royal Australasian College of Physicians.
6   C. Helman, *Suburban Shaman: Tales from medicine's front line*, Steele Roberts: Wellington, 2007.
7   New Zealand Medical Association, 'Consensus statement on the role of the doctor', *New Zealand Medical Journal*, vol. 124, 2011, pp. 117–20.
8   Complaints about medical practitioners comprised approximately 69% of complaints about any registered health practitioner to the Health and Disability Commissioner in the two years 1 July 2009 to 30 June 2011, with no other practitioner group comprising more than 8%. Personal communication, Office of the Health and Disability Commissioner, September 2011.
9   The word 'patient' is derived from the Latin 'patior', which means 'to suffer'.
10 Angela Coulter gives similar reasons in her John Fry lecture: A. Coulter, *The Autonomous Patient: Ending paternalism in medical care*, Nuffield Trust: London, 2002, pp. 6–8.
11 I recall the doctor who, on hearing the word 'consumer' used in the New Zealand Code of Health and Disability Services Consumers' Rights, protested: 'I *consume* toilet paper when I wipe my bum!' This crass comment was made during question time following my after-dinner speech to the Annual General Meeting of the Bay of Plenty branch of the New Zealand Medical Association, Tauranga, July 2001.

1   THE GOOD DOCTOR: THE IDEAL

1   General Medical Council, *Good Medical Practice*, London, 2006, para. 1.
2   D. Irvine, 'Everyone is entitled to a good doctor', *Medical Journal of Australia*, vol. 186, 2007, pp. 256–61 at p. 261.
3   A. Coulter, 'Patients' views of the good doctor', *British Medical Journal*, vol. 325, 2002, pp. 668–69 at p. 668.
4   The *New Zealand Herald* of 5 April 2011 carried the front-page headline 'Doctor signed up dead for cash', and detailed the disciplinary finding of 'professional misconduct' made against Dr Suresh Vatsyayann, who enrolled 44 patients (including four dead patients) at his practice without their knowledge, to obtain public funding. Yet patients defended him as 'an excellent doctor and a principled doctor' who provided free care to patients: A. Chambers, 'Doctor's wrongdoing', Letter to the editor, *New Zealand Herald*, 8 April 2011.
5   D. Galgut, *The Good Doctor*, Atlantic Books: London, 2003.
6   Roderigo a Castro, *Medicus Politicus*, 1614, quoted in A. Jonsen, *The New Medicine & the Old Ethics*, Harvard University Press: Cambridge, 1990, p. 24.
7   J. Groopman, *How Doctors Think*, Houghton Mifflin: Boston, 2007.
8   J. Rethans et al., 'The relationship between competence and performance: Implications for assessing practice performance', *Medical Education*, vol. 36, 2002, pp. 901–9.
9   See, for example, Health Quality & Safety Commission, *Making Our Hospitals Safer: Serious and sentinel events 2009/10*, Wellington, 2010.
10 N. Berlinger, *After Harm: Medical error and the ethics of forgiveness*, The Johns Hopkins University Press: Baltimore, 2005, p. xii.
11 Pharmacies were selected as a more neutral venue for soliciting patient opinions: M. Hutchinson and J. Reid, 'In the eyes of the Dunedin public, what constitutes professionalism in medicine?', *Journal of Primary Health Care*, vol. 3, 2011, pp. 10–15.
12 Quoted in Ministry of Health, *Training*

NOTES TO PAGES 4-11

the Medical Workforce 2006 and Beyond, Wellington, 2006, p. 5.

13 A. Old et al., 'Society's expectation of the role of the doctor in New Zealand: Results of a national survey', *New Zealand Medical Journal*, vol. 124, 2011, pp. 10–22.

14 J. Berger, *A Fortunate Man: The story of a country doctor*, Vintage Books: USA, 1997, p. 76.

15 D. Irvine, 'Patients, professionalism, and revalidation', *British Medical Journal*, vol. 330, 2005, pp. 1265–68 at p. 1265.

16 A. Chisholm, L. Cairncross and J. Askham, *Setting Standards: The views of members of the public and doctors on the standards of care and practice they expect of doctors*, Picker Institute Europe: Oxford, 2006.

17 This example is based on Health and Disability Commissioner, Case 08HDC03160, 18 June 2008 (unpublished), described in R. Paterson, 'Regulating for compassion?', *Journal of Law and Medicine*, vol. 18, 2010, pp. 58–67.

18 See S. Cartwright, *The Report of the Committee of Inquiry into Allegations Concerning the Treatment of Cervical Cancer at National Women's Hospital and into Other Related Matters*, Government Printing Office: Auckland, 1988.

19 Health and Disability Commissioner, *Liver biopsies for research performed during surgery without consent*, Case 00HDC07593, 30 August 2002, available at <http://www.hdc.org.nz/media/4746/00HDC07593casenote.pdf>.

20 S. Devi, 'US physicians urge end to unnecessary stent operations', *Lancet*, vol. 378, 2011, pp. 651–52. In a highly publicised decision, the Maryland Board of Physicians revoked the medical licence of leading interventional cardiologist Mark Midei, who was found to have inserted cardiac stents into arteries that didn't need them: *In the Matter of Mark G. Midei, MD, Respondent,* Maryland State Board of Physicians Final Decision and Order, 13 July 2011. The Board noted that 'pressure to perform' for his hospital employer appeared to be a factor in Dr Midei's unnecessary procedures.

21 See, for example, Health and Disability Commissioner, *Ophthalmologist, Dr C, Southland District Health Board*, Case 05HDC12122, 29 June 2007, available at <http://www.hdc.org.nz/media/14743/05hdc12122ophthalmologist.pdf>.

22 For an overview of the New Zealand Code and the complaints system, see R. Paterson, 'The patients' complaints system in New Zealand', *Health Affairs*, vol. 21, 2002, pp. 70–79. See also note 2 of the Preface to this book.

23 M. Stewart, 'Effective physician-patient communication and health outcomes: A review', *Canadian Medical Association Journal*, vol. 152, 1995, pp. 1423–33.

24 W. Levinson and P. Pizzo, 'Patient-physician communication. It's about time', *Journal of the American Medical Association*, vol. 305, 2011, pp. 1802–3 at p. 1802.

25 A. Coulter, *Engaging Patients in Healthcare*, Open University Press: Maidenhead, 2011.

26 M. Marshall and J. Bibby, 'Supporting patients to make the best decisions', *British Medical Journal*, vol. 342, 2011, p. d2117.

27 General Medical Council, *Consent: Patients and doctors making decisions together*, 2008, principle 2.

28 See, for example, Health and Disability Commissioner, *The Palms Medical Centre Ltd*, Case 08HDC06359, 30 June 2009.

29 Code of Health and Disability Services Consumers' Rights, right 1.

30 Code of Health and Disability Services Consumers' Rights, right 3.

31 United Kingdom Department of Health, *The NHS Constitution – The NHS belongs to us all*, London, 2009.

171

32 Some of my discussion of compassion, and the views of patients and doctors, is drawn from R. Paterson, 'Regulating for compassion?,' pp. 58–67.
33 Nationwide Health & Disability Consumer Advocacy Service, *The Art of Great Care: Stories from people who have experienced great care*, Auckland, 2010. The publication sought to respond to the backlash from some doctors, who claimed that patients would never be satisfied, and to strengthen consumer voice by sharing positive experiences.
34 Ibid., p. 7.
35 A. Broyard, *Intoxicated by My Illness: And other writings on life and death*, Clarkson Potter: New York, 1992, p. 45.
36 Ibid., p. 44.
37 'Fifteen Minutes after Gary Died', in R. Campo, *The Desire to Heal: A doctor's education in empathy, identity, and poetry*, W. W. Norton: New York, 1997, pp. 122–56.
38 J. Berger, *A Fortunate Man: The story of a country doctor*, Vintage Books: USA, 1997, p. 76.
39 There are many fine 'doctor as patient' books in which doctors narrate their unexpected journey as a patient, and the new insights they gained. In one example of this genre, Australian surgeon and rehabilitation specialist Tony Moore recounts his recovery from a horrific motor vehicle accident, and his new insights into illness and recovery, in *Cry of the Damaged Man: A personal journey of recovery*, Pan MacMillan Australia: Sydney, 1991.
40 A. Jonsen, *The New Medicine & the Old Ethics*, p. 24.
41 A. Fritsch, *Medicus Peccans*, Nuremberg, 1684, p. 2, cited in ibid., p. 24.
42 F. Peabody, 'The care of the patient', *Journal of the American Medical Association*, vol. 88, 1927, pp. 877–82 at p. 881.
43 Cited in C. Paul, 'A Question of Compassion', *New Zealand Listener*, 15 August 2009, pp. 33–34.
44 Cited in B. Lown, *The Lost Art of Healing: Practicing compassion in medicine*, Houghton Mifflin: Boston, 1996, p. xix.
45 Australian Medical Council, *Good Medical Practice: A code of conduct for doctors in Australia*, 2009, para. 1.4.
46 A. Jonsen, *The New Medicine & the Old Ethics*, p. 22.
47 Ibid., p. 23.
48 American Medical Association Code of Medical Ethics, 2001.
49 E. Freidson, *Profession of Medicine: A study of the sociology of applied knowledge*, The University of Chicago Press: Chicago, 1988.
50 S. Cruess, S. Johnston and R. Cruess, 'Professionalism for medicine: Opportunities and obligations', *Medical Journal of Australia*, vol. 177, 2002, pp. 208–11 at p. 210.
51 M. Dixon-Woods, K. Yeung and C. Bosk, 'Why is UK medicine no longer a self-regulating profession? The role of scandals involving "bad apple" doctors', *Social Science & Medicine*, vol. 73, 2011, pp. 1452–59 at pp. 1454, 1458.
52 D. Berwick, 'The epitaph of profession', *British Journal of General Practice*, vol. 59, 2009, pp. 128–31 at p. 130.
53 I. Kennedy, *Learning from Bristol: The report of the public inquiry into children's heart surgery at the Bristol Royal Infirmary 1984–1995*, Bristol Royal Infirmary Inquiry: United Kingdom, 2001, p. 201.
54 Personal recollection, Commonwealth Fund 10th Annual International Symposium on Health Care Policy, Washington DC, November 2007.
55 There were, however, some sceptics: K. Breen, 'Medical professionalism: Is it really under threat?', *Medical Journal of Australia*, vol. 186, 2007, pp. 596–98. Kerry Breen noted the need for broader community concerns to be taken into account, and pointed out that '[a]dditional initiatives that will assist the

community to trust and value medical professionalism in Australia include the increased expectation that all doctors will engage in continuing medical education and the establishment by medical boards of pathways to identify and assist poorly performing doctors': K. Breen, 'Medical Professionalism Project', *Medical Journal of Australia*, vol. 178, 2003, p. 93.

56 E. Campbell et al., 'Professionalism in medicine: Results of a national survey of physicians', *Annals of Internal Medicine*, vol. 147, 2007, pp. 795–802.

57 D. Irvine, 'Everyone is entitled to a good doctor', p. 256.

58 Medical Council of New Zealand, 'Statement on safe practice in an environment of resource limitation', Wellington, 2008, para. 4, available at <http://www.mcnz.org.nz/portals/0/Guidance/889358_MC_Statement%20Safe%20Practice%201_2_FA_WEB.pdf>.

59 S. Swensen et al., 'Cottage industry to postindustrial care – The revolution in health care delivery', *New England Journal of Medicine*, 20 January 2010, available at <http://www.nejm.org/doi/full/10.1056/NEJMp0911199>.

60 Ibid.

61 Ibid.

62 R. Veatch, *Patient, Heal Thyself: How the 'new medicine' puts the patient in charge*, Oxford University Press: New York, 2008.

63 R. Berkowitz et al., 'Improving disposition outcomes for patients in a geriatric skilled nursing facility', *Journal of the American Geriatrics Society*, vol. 59, 2011, pp. 1130–36.

64 A. Coulter and A. Collins, *Making Shared Decision-Making a Reality: No decision about me without me*, The King's Fund: London, 2011.

65 D. de Silva, *Helping People Help Themselves: A review of the evidence considering whether it is worthwhile to support self-management*, The Health Foundation: London, 2011.

66 W. Osler, 'The growth of a profession', *Canadian Journal of Medicine and Surgery*, vol. 14, 1885, p. 131, quoted in D. Irvine, 'Everyone is entitled to a good doctor', p. 261.

67 L. Donaldson, *Good Doctors, Safer Patients: Proposals to strengthen the system to assure and improve the performance of doctors and to protect the safety of patients. A report by the Chief Medical Officer*, Department of Health: London, 2006, para. 1, p. vi.

68 Ibid., para. 27, p. xi.

69 Personal recollection of statement by Arnold Milstein, The Commonwealth Fund and the Nuffield Trust, '7th International Meeting to Improve the Quality of Health Care: Strategies for Change and Action, 2005', Bagshot, England, July 2005.

2 PROBLEM DOCTORS: PART OF THE REALITY

1 R. Paterson, 'The public's hue and cry: Medical complaints in New Zealand', *Journal of Health Services Research & Policy*, vol. 6, 2001, pp. 193–94.

2 M. Bismark, T. Brennan, R. Paterson et al., 'Relationship between complaints and quality of care in New Zealand: A descriptive analysis of complainants and non-complainants following adverse events', *Quality & Safety in Health Care*, vol. 15, 2006, pp. 17–22.

3 W. Cunningham, 'The immediate and long-term impact on New Zealand doctors who receive patient complaints', *New Zealand Medical Journal*, vol. 117, 2004, available at <http://journal.nzma.org.nz/journal/117-1198/972/content.pdf>.

4 In the year ended 30 June 2010, only 36 investigations by the Health and Disability Commissioner (out of 1524 concluded complaints) resulted in

a breach finding against a provider; thus, only 2.4% of complaints were formally upheld: Health and Disability Commissioner, *Annual Report for the year ended 30 June 2010*, Auckland, 2010, pp. 6, 9.

5   M. Bismark, T. Brennan, R. Paterson et al., 'Relationship between complaints and quality of care in New Zealand', p. 22.

6   I am grateful to Fay Bishop, who laid the official complaint, for permission to retell her sister's story.

7   Health and Disability Commissioner, *General Practitioner, Dr B, General Practitioner, Dr C, An Accident and Medical Centre, Case 03HDC03134*, 28 June 2005, available at <http://www.hdc.org.nz/media/3020/03HDC03134gp.pdf>.

8   Ibid., p. 31. From a clinical governance perspective it was unacceptable for the medical centre to absolve itself from responsibility for ensuring adequate performance of its clinical staff. It is far better for problems in individual performance to be detected and addressed by fellow practitioners and managers in the practice setting, rather than wait for an external agency to become involved. The medical centre where Dr B worked provided no evidence of formal audit of his work or records, or that he was engaged in any peer review. In these circumstances, the centre was found vicariously liable for Dr B's breaches of the Code, since under section 72(3) of the Health and Disability Commissioner Act 1994, '[a]nything done or omitted by a person as the agent of an employing authority [such as a medical centre] shall ... be treated as done or omitted by that employing authority'.

9   A. Gawande, 'When good doctors go bad', *New Yorker*, 7 August 2000, pp. 60–69 at p. 63.

10 R. Smith, 'Preface', in P. Lens and G. van der Wal (eds), *Problem Doctors: A conspiracy of silence*, IOS Press: The Netherlands, 1997, p. vii.

11 P. Lens and G. van der Wal (eds), *Problem Doctors: A conspiracy of silence*, IOS Press: The Netherlands, 1997.

12 M. Rosenthal, *The Incompetent Doctor: Behind closed doors*, Open University Press: Buckingham, 1995.

13 M. Roland et al., 'Professional values and reported behaviours of doctors in the USA and UK: Quantitative survey', *British Medical Journal Quality & Safety*, 7 March 2011, available at <http://qualitysafety.bmj.com/content/early/2011/02/07/bmjqs.2010.048173.full.pdf>.

14 J. Smith, *The Shipman Inquiry*, The Stationery Office: Norwich, 2004, Fifth Report, para. 20.

15 Quoted in B. Hurwitz and A. Vass, 'What's a good doctor, and how can you make one?', *British Medical Journal*, vol. 325, 2002, pp. 667–68 at p. 667.

16 J. Smith, *The Shipman Inquiry*, Fifth Report, para. 79.

17 Ibid., para. 81.

18 Ibid., para. 26.3.

19 Ibid., para. 26.4.

20 Ibid., para. 26.203.

21 G. Davies, *Queensland Public Hospitals Commission of Inquiry Report 2005*, Queensland Health: Brisbane 2005, available at <http://www.qphci.qld.gov.au/final_report/Final_Report.pdf>.

22 Ibid., para. 1.2.

23 Ibid., para. 3.418(h), (k).

24 Dr Woodruff, quoted in ibid., para. 3.418(i).

25 H. Thomas, *Sick to Death: A manipulative surgeon and a healthy system in crisis – A disaster waiting to happen*, Allen & Unwin: New South Wales, 2007, is a journalist's gripping account of the saga of Dr Patel at Bundaberg Hospital. See also J. Dunbar, P. Reddy and S. May, *Deadly Healthcare*, Australian Academic Press: Queensland, 2011, for an academic critique of how a doctor with serious personality problems was able to exploit

26 A. Duffy, D. Barrett and M. Duggan, *Report of the Ministerial Inquiry into the Under-Reporting of Cervical Smear Abnormalities in the Gisborne Region*, Ministry of Health: Wellington, 2001, para. 5.36.

27 Patient A reached a confidential settlement with Dr Bottrill, after the Privy Council ruled that she was entitled to a retrial of her claim for exemplary damages. Although Patient A's medical misadventure was covered by accident compensation and she faced a statutory bar on claiming compensatory damages for negligence, the Privy Council concluded that exemplary damages may in rare cases be awarded, in the absence of intentional wrongdoing or conscious recklessness, 'where the defendant departed so far and so flagrantly from the dictates of ordinary or professional precepts of prudence, or standards of care': *A v Bottrill* [2003] 1 AC 449, para. 26.

28 A. Duffy, D. Barrett and M. Duggan, *Report of the Ministerial Inquiry into the Under-Reporting of Cervical Smear Abnormalities in the Gisborne Region*, para. 5.191.

29 Ibid., para. 5.190.

30 See P. Skegg, 'A fortunate experiment? New Zealand's experience with a legislated code of patients' rights', *Medical Law Review*, vol. 19, 2011, pp. 235–66; and T. Dare et al., 'Paternalism in practice: Informing patients about expensive unsubsidised drugs', *Journal of Medical Ethics*, vol. 36, 2010, pp. 260–64.

31 Health and Disability Commissioner Act 1994, s. 2(1).

32 J. Manning, 'Informed consent to medical treatment: The Common Law and New Zealand's code of patients' rights', *Medical Law Review*, vol. 12, 2004, pp. 181–216.

33 See P. Hartzband and J. Groopman, 'Untangling the web – patients, doctors, and the internet', *New England Journal of Medicine*, vol. 362, 2010, pp. 1063–66; and D. Rothman and D. Blumenthal (eds), *Medical Professionalism in the New Information Age*, Rutgers University Press: New Jersey, 2010.

34 The Commonwealth Fund, '2004 Commonwealth Fund International Health Policy Survey of Adults' Experiences with Primary Care', a telephone survey of 400 adults (18 years and over) in New Zealand, Australia, Canada and the United States, and 3061 adults in the United Kingdom. In the US and Canada, 56% and 40% of consumers wanted such information, compared with 28% in Australia and 24% in New Zealand. Intriguingly, only 18% of consumers in the UK wanted such information. More information about providers has become available to UK consumers since 2004, and it may be that expectations have risen in recent years.

35 Ibid. The range was 19% to 24%, with the United Kingdom reporting a better result of 13%.

36 Ibid. In New Zealand, 22% of surveyed adults who had seen a doctor in the past two years did not receive the results of a lab test or X-ray, or did not have the results clearly explained. The range was 16% to 28%.

37 Code of Health and Disability Services Consumers' Rights, right 4(5) states: 'Every consumer has the right to co-operation among providers to ensure quality and continuity of services.'

38 F. Frizelle, 'Informed consent – do less, talk more and write it all down', *New Zealand Medical Journal*, vol. 115, 2002, available at <http://journal.nzma.org.nz/journal/115-1162/181/content.pdf>.

39 P. Turner and C. Williams, 'Informed consent: Patients listen and read, but what information do they retain?', *New Zealand Medical Journal*, vol. 115, 2002, available at <http://journal.nzma.org.nz/journal/115-1164/218/content.pdf>.

40 A. Grubb, 'The doctor as fiduciary', *Current Legal Problems*, vol. 47, 1994, pp. 311–40.
41 Code of Health and Disability Services Consumers' Rights, clause 4.
42 K. Elkin et al., 'Doctors disciplined for professional misconduct in Australia and New Zealand, 2000–2009', *Medical Journal of Australia*, vol. 194, 2011, pp. 452–56.
43 Ibid.
44 Medical Council of New Zealand, *Sexual Boundaries in the Doctor–Patient Relationship: A resource for doctors*, Wellington, 2009, available at <http://www.mcnz.org.nz/portals/0/Publications/CO2563%20Sexual%20Boundaries%201_2_FA%20web.pdf>.
45 See, for example, *Director of Proceedings v Medical Practitioners Disciplinary Tribunal & Wiles* [2003] NZAR 250, in which the High Court stated: 'There can be no principle that every case of a sexual relationship between a doctor and patient must result in a disciplinary finding, each case must be judged on its facts' (Ellen France J, para. 50). In the District Court, Judge Lee described the Medical Council's 'zero tolerance' policy as exhibiting 'vestiges of a paternalistic attitude which sees women as childlike beings unable to think and act independently for themselves and needing protection for their own good' (District Court, Wellington, NA No. 69/01, 24 January 2002, Judge Lee, para. 49). Remarkably, the judge said that patients might see this as 'unjustified interference with their right as mature adults to live their lives as they see fit'! (para. 56).
46 This was the situation in *L v Robinson* [2000] 3 NZLR 499 (HC), where the patient recovered $50,000 in exemplary damages from her psychiatrist.
47 There is an extensive literature of physicians' conflicts of interest. For a comprehensive historical analysis of the development of medical practice in the United States until the late twentieth century, see M. Rodwin, *Medicine, Money, and Morals: Physicians' conflicts of interest*, Oxford University Press: New York, 1993. For a more recent discussion, see P. Hartzband and J. Groopman, 'Money and the changing culture of medicine', *New England Journal of Medicine*, vol. 360, 2009, pp. 101–3.
48 See case study on page 52.
49 See Code of Health and Disability Services Consumers' Rights, rights 9 and 6(1)(f).
50 S. Cartwright, *The Report of the Committee of Inquiry into Allegations Concerning the Treatment of Cervical Cancer at National Women's Hospital and into Other Related Matters*, Government Printing Office: Auckland, 1988. The *Report* has been contested in a revisionist history; see L. Bryder, *A History of the 'Unfortunate Experiment' at National Women's Hospital*, Auckland University Press: Auckland, 2009. But see J. Manning (ed.), *The Cartwright Papers: Essays on the Cervical Cancer Inquiry 1987–88*, Bridget Williams Books: Wellington, 2009, for a vigorous defence of the *Report*.
51 Health and Disability Commissioner, *Liver biopsies for research performed during surgery without consent*, Case 00HDC07593, 30 August 2002, available at <http://www.hdc.org.nz/media/4746/00HDC07593casenote.pdf>.
52 It was held that the neurologist had not communicated effectively with the patient about what was proposed, and had breached rights 5 and 9 of the Code: Health and Disability Commissioner, *Dr B (Neurosurgeon) and Dr C (Neurologist)*, Case 97HDC6996/JW, 20 October 1999, available at <http://www.hdc.org.nz/media/171800/97hdc6996.pdf>.
53 J. Stewart, *Blind Eye: How the medical establishment let a doctor get away with*

murder, Simon & Schuster: New York, 1999. The book is a riveting account of repeated regulatory failure enabling a psychopathic doctor to 'get away with murder' for over a decade. For readers interested in the phenomenon of medical murder, I recommend R. Kaplan, *Medical Murder: Disturbing cases of doctors who kill*, Allen & Unwin: New South Wales, 2009.

54 M. Scheikowski, 'Former doctor guilty of removing Carolyn DeWaegeneire's genitals without consent', *Daily Telegraph*, 10 March 2011.

55 Graeme Reeves was found guilty in July of assaulting two patients during internal pelvic examinations at his clinic. He was found not guilty of assaulting three other patients on similar sexual assault charges: 'Gynaecologist who mutilated patient jailed', *Guardian*, 1 July 2011, available at <http://www.guardian.co.uk/world/2011/jul/01/gynaecologist-mutilated-patient-jailed>.

56 'Croydon Day Surgery Hep C victims demand anaesthetist be charged', *Herald Sun*, 17 May 2011, available at <http://www.guardian.co.uk/world/2011/may/27/australian-doctor-charged-hepatitis-c>.

57 'Abortion clinic doctor charged with infecting patients with hepatitis C', *Guardian*, 27 May 2011.

58 Crimes Act 1961, s. 150A [my emphasis].

59 In the words of surgeon Ross Blair, quoted in 'Hell over for doctor', *New Zealand Herald*, 8 June 1995.

60 Current evidence suggests that there are higher rates of abuse of alcohol and other drugs in health professionals than in other groups of workers (Department of Health, *Invisible Patients: Report of the working group on the health of health professionals*, Department of Health: London, 2010, para. 2.8). Some researchers state that this perception is 'based more on folklore than on fact' (E. Weir, 'Substance abuse among physicians', *Canadian Medical Association Journal*, vol. 162, 2000, p. 1730).

61 P. O'Connor and A. Spickard, 'Physician impairment by substance abuse', *Medical Clinics of North America*, vol. 81, 1997, pp. 1037–52.

62 See New Zealand Health Practitioners Disciplinary Tribunal, Decision 154/Med07/80P, 8 May 2008, available at <http://www.hpdt.org.nz/portals/0/med078opfindings.pdf>; and *Dr A v Professional Conduct Committee* (HC, CIV-2008-404-2927, 5 September 2008, Keane J).

63 M. Bismark, E. Dauer, R. Paterson et al., 'Accountability sought by patients following adverse events from medical care: The New Zealand experience', *Canadian Medical Association Journal*, vol. 175, 2006, pp. 889–94.

64 Dean Williams, in answer to a question at the 3rd Annual National Medico-Legal Conference, Wellington, March 1995.

65 M. Bismark, E. Dauer, R. Paterson et al., 'Accountability sought by patients following adverse events from medical care'.

66 Under right 1 of New Zealand's Code of Health and Disability Services Consumers' Rights; and United Kingdom Department of Health, *The NHS Constitution – The NHS belongs to us all*, London, 2009.

67 Health and Disability Commissioner, Case 08HDC03160, 18 June 2008 (unpublished).

68 For a fuller discussion of the case, see R. Paterson, 'Regulating for compassion?', *Journal of Law and Medicine*, vol. 18, 2010, pp. 58–67 at pp. 64–65.

69 Health and Disability Commissioner, *General and Gastrointestinal Surgeon, Dr B, A District Health Board*, Case 09HDC01315, 22 January 2010, available at <http://www.hdc.org.nz/media/92402/09hdc01315surgeon.pdf>. The decision was widely debated in the media, with many commentators seeing it as a 'politically correct' ruling that would prevent doctors from

70 giving patients the 'home truths' they need to hear for the sake of their health. Several surgeons who discussed the case with me expressed a contrary view. They saw it as an unacceptable breach of professional standards that warranted discipline, and not merely the communication skills training that I recommended.
70 Medical Council of New Zealand, 'Unprofessional behaviour and the health care team. Protecting patient safety', Wellington, 2009, available at <http://www.mcnz.org.nz/portals/0/Publications/Unprofessional_behaviour.pdf>.
71 Health and Disability Commissioner, *Dr Roman Hasil and Whanganui District Health Board, 2005–2006*, Auckland, 2008.

3 THE ROADBLOCKS: WHY IS CHANGE SO DIFFICULT?

1 In New Zealand, the Health and Disability Commissioner Act 1994 provides for publicly funded, independent health and disability services consumer advocates to 'act as an advocate for health consumers and disability services consumers', s. 30(a).
2 In November 2008, in a clear signal to the medical profession, New Zealand's Minister of Health, Tony Ryall, publicly committed to this move within 24 hours of assuming the health portfolio. It won him immediate plaudits from medical professional organisations, as it was seen to be supportive of self-regulation.
3 Information supplied by the New Zealand Medical Association, August 2011.
4 See the blunt language of Judge Rod Joyce QC in *Beaumont-Connop v Waitemata Health Ltd* (District Court, North Shore, NP No. 1079/01, 25 October 2002), paras 230 and 92, dismissing a family's negligence claim against a hospital.
5 Press release, General Medical Council, 'Record number of complaints and disciplinary hearings against doctors', 24 October 2011, available at <http://www.gmc-uk.org/news/10785.asp>.
6 Research undertaken in 2010, by TNS for the Medical Council of New Zealand (*NZ Medical Consumer Research*), found that 75% of 523 survey respondents (members of the public) said their confidence in doctors would be increased if they knew that doctors' performance was subject to a regular review. A survey in England in 2005, conducted by Mori Social Research on behalf of the Department of Health (*Attitudes to Medical Regulation and Revalidation of Doctors: Research among the general public, GPs and hospital doctors*), found that half those surveyed assumed regular checks of doctors' competence already occurred; 90% thought such checks were important.
7 J. Robinson, *A Patient Voice at the GMC: A lay member's view of the General Medical Council*, Health Rights: London, 1988, p. 41.
8 J. Robinson, 'The Price of Deceit: The Reflections of an Advocate', in M. Rosenthal, L. Mulcahy and S. Lloyd-Bostock (eds), *Medical Mishaps: Pieces of the puzzle*, Open University Press: Buckingham, 1999, ch. 22, pp. 246–56.
9 Carl Elliott notes the role of pharmaceutical companies in deciding which health issues appear to have 'grass-roots patient support' (*Better Than Well: American medicine meets the American Dream*, W. W. Norton: New York, 2003, p. 125).
10 A recent New Zealand example was the successful campaign by the *Otago Daily Times* and the *Southland Times*, supported by local citizens who joined in street marches, to prevent the closure of the neurosurgery service at Dunedin

Hospital. For a US example, read the account of the ultimately unsuccessful battle to save Winchendon Hospital in Massachusetts, told in M. Gerteis et al. (eds), *Through the Patient's Eyes: Understanding and promoting patient-centered care*, Jossey-Bass: San Francisco, 1993.

11   See J. Manning, 'Priority-setting processes for medicines: The United Kingdom, Australia and New Zealand', *Journal of Law and Medicine*, vol. 18, 2011, pp. 439–52. As Manning notes, this funding episode mirrored a similar Australian experience in relation to Herceptin in 2000.

12   M. Marshall and J. Braspenning, 'European family practice and public accountability', *Family Practice*, 2001, vol. 18, pp. 473–74 at p. 473.

13   P. Shekelle et al., *Does Public Release of Performance Results Improve Quality of Care? A systematic review*, The Health Foundation: London, 2008. See also M. Marshall et al., 'The public release of performance data: What do we expect to gain? A review of the evidence', *Journal of the American Medical Association*, vol. 283, 2000, pp. 1866–74.

14   J. Hyatt, 'Let's welcome the early symptoms of social health', *Guardian*, 2 June 2011.

15   O. O'Neill, *A Question of Trust*, Cambridge University Press: Cambridge, 2002, p. 87.

16   R. Tallis, *Hippocratic Oaths: Medicine and its discontents*, Atlantic Books: London, 2004, p. 103.

17   M. Millenson, *Demanding Medical Excellence: Doctors and accountability in the information age*, The University of Chicago Press: Chicago, 1997, p. 3.

18   Ibid., p. 312.

19   Harris Interactive poll, January 2011; results summary available at <http://blog.insiderpages.com/2011/01/13/do-you-think-more-about-technology-than-your-health/>.

20   D. Williams, 'More performance data to be released under new transparency guidelines', *Health Service Journal*, 2 June 2011, available at <http://www.hsj.co.uk/news/primary-care/more-performance-data-to-be-released-under-new-transparency-guidelines/5030478.article>.

21   Public Law 111–148—March 23 2010, 124 STAT. 967, s. 10331, Public reporting of performance information. From January 2013, the published information is to include 'information on physician performance that provides comparable information for the public on quality and patient experience measures with respect to physicians enrolled in the Medicare program'. Physicians whose performance on measures is being publicly reported are to be given a 'reasonable opportunity . . . to review [their] individual results before they are made public'.

22   There have been periodic attempts by New Zealand consumer groups to push this agenda: see, for example, the paper on 'Fitness to practice' by former Women's Health Action trustee Judi Strid, presented at the Medical Council of New Zealand 'Fitness to practice' seminar, Wellington, May 1999, available at <http://www.womens-health.org.nz/index.php?page=fitness-to-practice>.

23   I. Allen, 'Doctors under stress', *British Medical Association News*, 10 April 1996, pp. 32–34, cited in R. Tallis, *Hippocratic Oaths*, p. 66.

24   D. Mechanic, 'Physician discontent. Challenges and opportunities', *Journal of the American Medical Association*, vol. 290, 2003, pp. 941–46.

25   C. Joyce et al., 'Australian doctors' satisfaction with their work: Results from the MABEL longitudinal survey of doctors', *Medical Journal of Australia*, vol. 194, 2011, pp. 30–33.

26   A. Zuger, 'Dissatisfaction with medical practice', *New England Journal of Medicine*, vol. 350, 2004, pp. 69–75. Zuger argues the golden age of medicine in the

mid-twentieth century was an aberration and that dissatisfaction within the medical profession has a long vintage.
27 D. Mechanic, 'Physician discontent. Challenges and opportunities'.
28 L. Beecham, 'BMA Chairman criticises erosion of clinical autonomy', *British Medical Journal*, vol. 327, 2003, p. 8.
29 V. Harpwood, *Medicine, Malpractice and Misapprehensions*, Routledge-Cavendish: Abingdon, 2007, ch. 5, pp. 130–62.
30 R. Boswell, 'E Pluribus Unum', *Medspeak*, The Newsletter of the New Zealand Medical Association, June 2005, p. 2.
31 K. Breen, 'Medical professionalism: Is it really under threat?', *Medical Journal of Australia*, vol. 186, 2007, pp. 596–98 at p. 597.
32 R. Tallis, *Hippocratic Oaths: Medicine and its discontents*, Atlantic Books: London, 2004.
33 Ibid., p. 41.
34 Burnout appears common among practising doctors, with rates ranging from 25% to 60% (T. Shanafelt et al., 'Burnout and self-reported patient care in an internal medicine residency program', *Annals of Internal Medicine*, vol. 136, 2002, pp. 358–67).
35 R. Smith, 'Why are doctors so unhappy?', *British Medical Journal*, vol. 322, 2001, pp. 1073–74.
36 Health Practitioners Competence Assurance Act 2003, s. 3(1).
37 Ross Blair, quoted in 'More controls, slower delivery warns health expert', *Marlborough Express*, 9 May 2003.
38 O. O'Neill, *A Question of Trust*, Cambridge University Press: Cambridge, 2002, p. 57.
39 Ibid., p. 50.
40 Ibid., p. 58 [emphasis in original].
41 R. Mannion and H. Davies, 'Payment for performance in health care', *British Medical Journal*, vol. 336, 2008, pp. 306–8.
42 S. Iliffe and J. Munro, 'General practitioners and incentives', *British Medical Journal*, vol. 307, 1993, pp. 1156–57.
43 Compare R. Smith, 'Why are doctors so unhappy?'.
44 M. Stacey, *Regulating British Medicine: The General Medical Council*, John Wiley & Sons: Chichester, 1992, p. 203.
45 C. Ameringer, *State Medical Boards and the Politics of Public Protection*, The Johns Hopkins University Press: Baltimore, 1999.
46 Ibid., p. 104.
47 I use the phrase 'co-regulatory' agency to describe a body, such as the New Zealand Health and Disability Commissioner, which shares responsibility for regulating health practitioners with health practitioner boards. New South Wales has also been described as having a system of co-regulation of the medical profession: D. Thomas, 'New South Wales: The Complaints Unit/Health Care Complaints Commission', in D. Thomas (ed.), *Medicine Called to Account: Health complaints mechanisms in Australia*, University of New South Wales: Sydney, 2003, p. 28.
48 The Health Practitioner Regulation National Law Act 2009, s. 3(2)(a).
49 G. Davies, *Queensland Public Hospitals Commission of Inquiry Report*, 2005, para. 3.136.
50 Ibid., para. 6.448.
51 Health and Disability Commissioner, *Tauranga Hospitals Inquiry, Case 04HDC07920*, 18 February 2005, available at <http://www.hdc.org.nz/media/3114/04HDC07920surgeon.pdf>.
52 Health and Disability Commissioner, *Dr Roman Hasil and Whanganui District Health Board, 2005–2006*, Auckland, 2008.
53 A. Reid, 'To Discipline or Not To Discipline? Managing Poorly Performing Doctors', in I. Freckelton (ed.), *Regulating Health Practitioners*, The Federation Press: Sydney, 2005, pp. 91–112; and I. St George, 'Assessing performance 1: There but for the Grace of God go I', *New Zealand Family*

Physician, vol. 31, 2004, pp. 45–47.
54 Council for Healthcare Regulatory Excellence, *Performance Review of the Medical Council of New Zealand: Promoting improvement in regulation through international collaboration*, London, 2010, paras 7.26–7.27. It would probably help address perceptions of cosiness with the profession if the Chair of the Medical Council was not a former Chair of the New Zealand Medical Association, as two of the three Council chairs have been in the past ten years.
55 Ibid., paras 7.31, 9.8.
56 D. Irvine, *The Doctor's Tale. Professionalism and Public Trust*, Radcliffe Medical Press: Abingdon, 2003.
57 Quoted in A. Mostrous, 'Shipman judge "in despair" over doctors who are not struck off', *The Times*, 4 November 2011.
58 'Face the Facts: Doctors in the Dock', BBC Radio 4, 3 February 2001, available at <http://www.bbc.co.uk/programmes/b00y2vgh>.
59 For a fascinating ethnographic study of the implementation of the new law at three US hospitals, see K. Kellogg, *Challenging Operations. Medical Reform and Resistance in Surgery*, The University of Chicago Press: Chicago, 2011.
60 See R. Smith, '"Regulating" doctors: what makes them practise as they do?', in *The quest for excellence: What is good health care? Essays in honour of Robert J. Maxwell*, The King's Fund: London, 1998, pp. 109–31.
61 R. Tallis, *Hippocratic Oaths*, p. 185.
62 D. Irvine, *The Doctor's Tale*, p. 198.
63 J. Robinson, 'The price of deceit: reflections of an advocate', in M. Rosenthal, L. Mulcahy and S. Lloyd-Bostock (eds), *Medical Mishaps*, ch. 22, p. 254.
64 C. Paul, 'Internal and external morality of medicine: Lessons from New Zealand', *British Medical Journal*, vol. 320, 2000, pp. 499–503.
65 For a sympathetic account of medical graduates swearing the Hippocratic Oath, see H. Markel, '"I Swear by Apollo" – On taking the Hippocratic Oath', *New England Journal of Medicine*, vol. 350, 2004, pp. 2026–28 at p. 2028. Some bioethicists (notably Robert Veatch) question its relevance and appropriateness.
66 Interestingly, there is anecdotal evidence that doctors may be more willing to judge an 'outsider', such as an overseas-trained doctor. Rosenthal makes this point in *The Incompetent Doctor* (p. 99) and it accords with my observation of cases of medico-legal processes in New Zealand. In the campaign in the mid-1990s to change the threshold for 'medical manslaughter' in New Zealand, it was the prosecution of a locally trained anaesthetist (following earlier cases involving overseas-trained anaesthetists) that galvanised the medical profession.
67 As anaesthetist Steven Bolsin found after he blew the whistle on problems at Bristol Royal Infirmary, even though his actions were validated in the subsequent public inquiry: see T. Faunce et al., 'When silence threatens safety: Lessons from the first Canberra Hospital Neurosurgical Inquiry', *Journal of Law and Medicine*, vol. 12, 2004, pp. 112–18.
68 Personal recollection, meeting with Royal Australasian College of Surgeons New Zealand officials, April 2004. It took an anaesthetist colleague to have the courage to make the complaint to hospital management that led to the surgeon's suspension.
69 I. Kennedy, *Learning from Bristol: The Report of the Public Inquiry into children's heart surgery at the Bristol Royal Infirmary 1984–1995*, Bristol Royal Infirmary Inquiry: United Kingdom, 2001, p. 201.
70 See D. Chisholm, 'The disappearing white male doctor', *North & South*, September 2010, pp. 40–52.
71 In 2010, international medical graduates

comprised 41.1% of the medical workforce in New Zealand: New Zealand Medical Council, *The New Zealand Medical Workforce in 2010*, Wellington, 2011.
72 See R. Smith, '"Regulating" doctors', p. 111.
73 The classic account of the process of socialisation of young surgical trainees is by American sociologist Charles Bosk, in *Forgive and Remember: Managing medical failure*, The University of Chicago Press: Chicago, 1979. Bosk observes a hospital to be 'a training institution charged with the socialization of recruits' (p. 177).
74 J. Robinson, 'The Price of Deceit: Reflections of an Advocate', in M. Rosenthal, L. Mulcahy and S. Lloyd-Bostock (eds), *Medical Mishaps*, ch. 22, p. 252.
75 P. Malpas, 'Reflecting on senior medical students' ethics reports at the University of Auckland', *Journal of Medical Ethics*, vol. 37, 2011, pp. 627–30.
76 M. Rosenthal, *The Incompetent Doctor: Behind closed doors*, Open University Press: Buckingham, 1995, p. 96.
77 N. McIntyre and K. Popper, 'The critical attitude in medicine: The need for a new ethics', *British Medical Journal*, vol. 287, 1983, pp. 1919–23.
78 See D. Collins and C. Brown, 'The impact of the Cartwright Report upon the regulation, discipline and accountability of medical practitioners in New Zealand', *Journal of Law and Medicine*, vol. 16, 2009, pp. 595–613.
79 Simply being subject to a complaint may induce a sense of shame: see W. Cunningham, 'The immediate and long-term impact on New Zealand doctors who receive patient complaints', *New Zealand Medical Journal*, vol. 117, 2004, available at <http://journal.nzma. org.nz/journal/117-1198/972/content. pdf>; see also W. Cunningham and H. Wilson, 'Complaints, shame and defensive medicine', *British Medical Journal Quality & Safety*, vol. 20, 2011, pp. 449–52.
80 Health and Disability Commissioner, *Capital and Coast District Health Board, Case 05HDC11908*, 22 March 2007, available at <http://www.hdc.org.nz/media/14834/05hdc11908dhb.pdf>. The report was a catalyst for improvements at hospitals around the country, particularly in systems for responding to physiologically unstable patients.
81 P. Roberts, 'Loyal to the profession of medicine and just and generous to its members', New Zealand Medical Association Presidential Address 2007.
82 R. Paterson, 2008 Nordmeyer lecture, *Inquiries into Health Care: Learning or lynching?*, University of Otago: Wellington, 2008, pp. 11–13.
83 I acknowledge the minority of doctors from all specialties who provide inquiry bodies with expert advice, recognising this as a form of public service. Furthermore, whereas in the past patients often encountered a wall of professional resistance, this is changing, and some medical experts are willing to provide patients with advice to pursue a complaint or claim.
84 McIntyre and Popper noted that 'in the search for mistakes there should be no denigration of others nor any condemnation associated with the process of peer review' ('The critical attitude in medicine: The need for a new ethics', p. 1922).
85 C. Paul and L. Holloway, 'No new evidence on the cervical cancer study', *New Zealand Medical Journal*, vol. 103, 1990, pp. 581–83 at p. 583.
86 J. Smith, *The Shipman Inquiry*, The Stationery Office: Norwich, 2004, Fifth Report, para. 79.
87 G. Currie, J. Waring and R. Finn, 'The limits of knowledge management for UK public sector modernization: The case of patient safety and service quality', *Public Administration*, vol. 86, 2008, pp. 363–85 at p. 377. The quote is

from a consultant anaesthetist, following a dispute with a consultant surgeon after submitting an incident report implicating his practice.
88 This criticism is levelled at the medical profession in R. Gibson and J. Singh, *Wall of Silence: The untold story of the medical mistakes that kill and injure millions of Americans*, LifeLine Press: Washington DC, 2003, ch. 8, pp. 135–54.
89 C. Bosk, *Forgive and Remember*, p. 191.
90 A. Gawande, *Complications: A surgeon's notes on an imperfect science*, Profile Books: London, 2002, p. 60.
91 This is consistent with the model of M & M described in New South Wales Department of Health, *The Clinician's Toolkit for Improving Patient Care*, New South Wales, 2001, pp. 28–30. Some New Zealand hospitals hold several combined medical and surgical M & M meetings each year, to promote a common systems-focused approach (personal communication, Dr Mary Seddon, December 2011).
92 M. Rosenthal, *The Incompetent Doctor: Behind closed doors*, Open University Press: Buckingham, 1995.
93 It is difficult to resist the obvious observation that this is a 'double whammy': only members of the profession can judge, but they are highly reluctant to do so!
94 H. Thomas, *Sick to Death: A manipulative surgeon and a healthy system in crisis – A disaster waiting to happen*, Allen & Unwin: New South Wales, 2007, p. 218. See discussion on pages 37–39.
95 M. Rosenthal, *The Incompetent Doctor*, pp. 4–5. The 'Blue Book' was the official guidance on professional conduct and discipline published by the General Medical Council from 1963 to 1993.
96 GfK NOP Social Research, *Research into Fitness for Practise Referrals 2011*, General Medical Council: London, 2011.
97 Medical Council of New Zealand, *What to do when you have concerns about a colleague*, Wellington, 2010.
98 Compare s. 34(1) (mandatory reporting of health concerns) with s. 45(1), (2) (authorised reporting of competence concerns) of the Health Practitioners Competence Assurance Act 2003.
99 Right 4(2) of the Code of Health and Disability Services Consumers' Rights [my emphasis].
100 Health Practitioner Regulation National Law Act 2009, ss. 140, 141.
101 See, generally, Senate Finance and Public Administration References Committee, *The Administration of Health Practitioner Registration by the Australian Health Practitioner Regulation Agency*, Commonwealth of Australia: Canberra, 2011, pp. 100–3. The former President of the Australian Medical Association submitted that '[c]ombined with the subjective test intrinsic to the notion of "reasonable belief", the threshold for the requirement of triggering notification is low' (para. 5.47).
102 The test derives from the judgment of McNair J in *Bolam v Friern Hospital Management Committee* [1957] 1 WLR 582. The case and the subsequent tendency of judges to 'Bolamise' or give undue deference to medical opinion is analysed by J. Miola, *Medical Ethics and Medical Law. A Symbiotic Relationship*, Hart Publishing: Oxford, 2007, pp. 9–14.
103 *Bolitho v City & Hackney Health Authority* [1998] AC 232. The extent of the *Bolitho* qualification is discussed in M. Brazier and J. Miola, 'Bye-Bye Bolam: A medical litigation revolution?', *Medical Law Review*, vol. 8, 2000, pp. 85–114.
104 The Australian reforms are analysed in B. Bennett and I. Freckelton, 'Life after the Ipp reforms: Medical negligence law', in I. Freckelton and K. Petersen, *Disputes & Dilemmas in Health Law*, The Federation Press: Sydney, 2006, pp. 381–405.
105 As required by right 4(1) of the Code of Health and Disability Services Consumers' Rights.

106 See D. Wong and R. Paterson, 'Commissioner's Comment: Ovarian cancer and expert advice', *New Zealand Family Physician*, vol. 32, 2005, pp. 50–52.

107 Health and Disability Commissioner, *Death by cardiac arrest following transfer of care, Case 99HDC10975*, 27 June 2000, available at <http://www.hdc.org.nz/media/5090/99HDC10975casenote.pdf>.

108 R. Goldman, 'The reliability of peer assessments of quality of care', *Journal of the American Medical Association*, vol. 267, 1992, pp. 958–60. Goldman examined the literature regarding the inter-reviewer reliability of the standard practice of peer assessment of quality of care, and concluded that '[o]verall, physician agreement regarding quality of care is only slightly better than the level expected by chance' (p. 958).

109 The perception that poor-quality testimony by physicians is prevalent is leading to an increase in extrajudicial regulation in the United States: see A. Kesselheim and D. Studdert, 'Role of professional organizations in regulating physician expert witness testimony', *Journal of the American Medical Association*, vol. 298, 2007, pp. 2907–9.

110 Advocates and lawyers for patients claim that enhanced scrutiny of physician expert witnesses unfairly targets experts on the plaintiff's side, contributing to a 'conspiracy of silence': see ibid., p. 2907.

111 R. Godbold and A. McCallin, 'Setting the standard? New Zealand's approach to ensuring health and disability services of an appropriate standard', *Journal of Law and Medicine*, vol. 13, 2005, pp. 125–34.

112 See R. Kaplan, K. Posner and F. Cheney, 'Effect of outcome on physician judgments of appropriateness of care', *Journal of the American Medical Association*, vol. 265, 1991, pp. 1957–60; and K. Hendriksen and H. Kaplan, 'Hindsight bias, outcome knowledge and adaptive learning', *Quality and Safety in Health Care*, vol. 12, suppl. 2, 2003, pp. ii46–ii50.

113 My comments in this section are drawn from R. Paterson, 2008 Nordmeyer lecture, *Inquiries into Health Care*, pp. 1–25.

114 In New Zealand, this is a legacy of the Privy Council's overturning of Justice Peter Mahon's Erebus Inquiry report (for breach of natural justice in making the 'litany of lies' comment that had not been put to Air New Zealand). P. Mahon, *Report of the Royal Commission to inquire into the Crash on Mount Erebus, Antarctica, of a DC10 Aircraft operated by Air New Zealand Ltd*, Government Printer: Wellington, 1981; *Re Erebus Royal Commission; Air New Zealand Ltd v Mahon* [1983] NZLR 662.

115 *Royal Australasian College of Surgeons v Phipps* [1999] 3 NZLR 1, p. 12 (Court of Appeal).

116 G. Davies, *Queensland Public Hospitals Commission of Inquiry Report*, para. 3.376.

117 New Zealand District Health Boards Senior Medical and Dental Officers' Collective Agreement 1 July 2007 until 30 April 2010 (varied as at 9 September 2010), clause 42, 'Investigations of Clinical Practice'.

118 Health and Disability Commissioner, *Tauranga Hospitals Inquiry, Case 04HDC07920*, 18 February 2005, p. 41.

119 *Royal Australasian College of Surgeons v Phipps* [1999] 3 NZLR 1, p. 12 (Court of Appeal), citing the leading case of *Durayappah v Fernando* [1967] 2 ACC 337 at p. 349 (Privy Council).

120 Health and Disability Commissioner, *Tauranga Hospitals Inquiry, Case 04HDC07920*, p. 40.

121 *Air New Zealand v Samu* [1994] 1 ERNZ 93, p. 95.

122 Personal recollection from conversations with DHB chief executives.

123 Michael Ludbrook, chairman of Southern Cross Norfolk Hospital, quoted in L. Andrews, 'Medical panel "keeping public in dark"', *Bay of Plenty Times*, 6 December 2003.

124 Health and Disability Commissioner, *Dr Roman Hasil and Whanganui District Health Board, 2005–2006*, Auckland, 2008, pp. 85–86.

125 I make this point in relation to the initial determination whether a doctor breached their duty of care to a patient. In most common law systems, a patient who brings a civil claim in negligence will face the additional hurdle of proving causation, i.e., that the breach caused harm.

126 Health and Disability Commissioner, *Tauranga Hospitals Inquiry*, Case 04HDC07920.

127 See *DPP v P* [1991] 2 AC 447 (House of Lords) and *R v Holtz* [2003] 1 NZLR 667 (Court of Appeal) for a general statement of this principle in criminal proceedings.

128 In *Applebee v Alsaffar* [2011] TASSC 1, the Supreme Court of Tasmania held that evidence of a surgeon's tendency to proceed with total gall bladder removal operations when unable to view the common bile duct, thereby risking damage to ductal structures, was relevant to a claim of negligence for proceeding with an operation in similar circumstances.

129 In New Zealand, 'protected quality assurance activities' and participants therein are protected under the Health Practitioners Competence Assurance Act 2003, ss. 52–63.

130 Ibid., s. 52.

131 Ibid., s. 58(1)(e), (2).

132 Judge Graham Hubble in *Parry v Medical Practitioners Disciplinary Tribunal* (District Court, Auckland, 30 May 2001), para. 85.

133 M. Johnston, 'The many trials of Dr Parry', *New Zealand Herald*, 30 October 2004. There was certainly a major injustice to Dr Parry in the decision of a parliamentary select committee to hold its own inquiry, effectively sitting as a 'kangaroo court' outside of established processes.

134 H. Cull, *Review of Processes Concerning Adverse Medical Events*, Ministry of Health: Wellington, 2001.

135 Ibid., p. 72.

136 Ibid., p. 73. Cull noted the findings of the Parliamentary Committee on the Healthcare Complaints Commission of New South Wales in its report *Mandatory Reporting of Medical Negligence* (2000) that '[c]entralised knowledge of medical negligence litigation information by regulatory bodies is extremely important' (p. 10).

137 As Health and Disability Commissioner, I opposed the proposal that HDC be the central repository of information about a practitioner, arguing that health practitioner registration boards are the logical agencies to hold all information about a practitioner's track record (including complaint, health, competence or conduct information).

138 See M. Bismark et al., 'Claiming behaviour in a no-fault system of medical injury: A descriptive analysis of claimants and non-claimants', *Medical Journal of Australia*, vol. 185, 2006, pp. 203–7.

139 Accident Compensation Act 2001, s. 284.

140 D. Studdert and T. Brennan, 'No-fault compensation for medical injuries: The prospect for error prevention', *Journal of the American Medical Association*, vol. 286, 2001, pp. 217–23 at p. 219.

141 J. Manning, 'New Zealand's remedial response to adverse events in healthcare', *Torts Law Journal*, vol. 16, 2008, pp. 120–55 at p. 147.

142 Ibid., p. 148.

143 Information supplied by ACC, July 2011. In the early years of the treatment injury provisions, ACC declined to provide

names of individual practitioners when making a risk report to a registration board, leaving boards in an impossible situation. Practitioner names are now provided.
144 Letter from Chief Executive of ACC to author as Health and Disability Commissioner, 30 May 2007.
145 M. Mello et al., '"Health courts" and accountability for patient safety', *Milbank Quarterly*, vol. 84, 2006, pp. 459–92.

4 PRESCRIPTION FOR CHANGE: WHAT CAN WE IMPROVE?

1 Society for Cardiothoracic Surgery in Great Britain & Ireland, *Maintaining Patients' Trust: Modern medical professionalism*, Dentrite Clinical Systems: Henley-on-Thames, 2011.
2 TNS Social Research, *Awareness, Trust and Information: Research with New Zealand medical consumers*, Medical Council of New Zealand: Wellington, 2007.
3 Council for Healthcare Regulatory Excellence, *Performance Review of the Medical Council of New Zealand: Promoting improvement in regulation through international collaboration*, London, 2010, para. 3.13. When the same questions were asked in 2010, the results were marginally better: 12% of the public thought that doctors in general were 'very trustworthy', compared with 44% holding that opinion of their own doctor; 6% of respondents thought their own doctor 'very untrustworthy' (TNS New Zealand, *NZ Medical Consumer Research*, Medical Council of New Zealand: Auckland, 2010, slide 24).
4 TNS New Zealand, *NZ Medical Consumer Research*, slide 34.
5 M. Marshall, 'Revalidation: A professional imperative', *British Journal of General Practice*, vol. 59, 2009, pp. 476–77 at p. 476.
6 Ibid.
7 C. Chantler and R. Ashton, 'The purpose and limits to professional self-regulation', *Journal of the American Medical Association*, vol. 302, 2009, pp. 2032–33 at p. 2033.
8 Department of Health, *Enabling Excellence: Autonomy and accountability for healthcare workers, social workers and social care workers*, The Stationery Office: London, 2011, p. 4.
9 P. Shekelle et al., *Does Public Release of Performance Results Improve Quality of Care? A Systematic Review*, The Health Foundation: London, 2008.
10 I am indebted to Justin Oakley for his clear exposition of the arguments in S. Clarke and J. Oakley (eds), *Informed Consent and Clinical Accountability: The ethics of report cards on surgeon performance*, Cambridge University Press: Cambridge, 2007.
11 N. Tomes, 'The "Information Rx"', in D. Rothman and D. Blumenthal (eds), *Medical Professionalism in the New Information Age*, Rutgers University Press, New Jersey, 2010, pp. 40–65 at pp. 61, 64.
12 S. Holt and R. Paterson, 'Medico-legal secrecy in New Zealand', *Journal of Law and Medicine*, vol. 15, 2008, pp. 602–25.
13 S. Cartwright, *The Report of the Committee of Inquiry into Allegations Concerning the Treatment of Cervical Cancer at National Women's Hospital and into Other Related Matters*, Government Printing Office: Auckland, 1988, p. 172 [emphasis added].
14 Health and Disability Commissioner, *Naming Providers in Public HDC Reports*, 2008, p. 11, available at <http://www.hdc.org.nz/media/18311/naming%20providers%20in%20public%20hdc%20reports.pdf>.
15 Ibid., pp. 4–5.
16 J. Manning, 'Health Care Law – Part 1: Common Law Developments', *New Zealand Law Review*, vol. 181, 2004, pp. 181–213 at p. 206.

17 In relation to consumer reliance on public registers being up to date, see 'How do consumers know they are engaging with a competent health practitioner?', *Women's Health Update*, vol. 15, 2011, p. 4.
18 Unsurprisingly, physicians and hospitals, and their attorneys, may seek to circumvent reporting requirements – for example, by capping settlements just below the amount that triggers notification.
19 Personal communication, Chair, NHS Litigation Authority, October 2011.
20 In 2001, the Health Select Committee of the New South Wales Parliament recommended mandatory reporting of malpractice claims data but, predictably, no change ensued: Committee on the Health Care Complaints Commission, *Report on Mandatory Reporting of Medical Negligence*, Parliament of New South Wales: Sydney, 2000.
21 Videoconference with Martin Erichsen, head of the Danish Patient Insurance Association, and New Zealand stakeholders during ACC treatment injury reform process, Wellington, 2003.
22 M. Mello, A. Kachalia and D. Studdert, *Administrative Compensation for Medical Injuries: Lessons from three foreign systems*, The Commonwealth Fund: New York, 2011, p. 7.
23 Agreement between the Health and Disability Commissioner and the Medical Council of New Zealand, April 2009.
24 M. Bismark, M. Spittal and D. Studdert, 'Prevalence and characteristics of complaint-prone doctors in private practice in Victoria', *Medical Journal of Australia*, vol. 195, 2011, pp. 25–28.
25 Less than 4% of complaints to the Health and Disability Commissioner result in a formal investigation: Health and Disability Commissioner, *Annual Report for the year ended 30 June 2010*, Auckland, 2010, p. 6. This is consistent with the approach taken by most Australian healthcare complaint commissions.
26 <http://www.consumerreports.org/health/doctors-hospitals/your-doctor-relationship/how-to-choose-a-doctor/how-to-check-credentials/how-to-check-credentials.htm>.
27 E. Stone et al., *Accessing Physician Information on the Internet*, The Commonwealth Fund: New York, 2002.
28 See <http://www.health.govt.nz/yourhealth-topics/health-care-services/visiting-doctor>.
29 Statements made on public release of report of the Council for Healthcare Regulatory Excellence, *Performance Review of the Medical Council of New Zealand: Promoting improvement in regulation through international collaboration*, in October 2010.
30 L. Priest, 'How do I do a background check on my doctor?', *Globe and Mail*, 27 March 2011.
31 M. Larson et al., 'Survey of State Medical and Osteopathy Board disciplinary web sites in 2006', *Health Matrix*, vol. 19, 2009, pp. 1–16.
32 D. Wilson, 'Obama administration removes disciplinary files from the web', *New York Times*, 15 September 2011.
33 Ministry of Health, *Review of the Health Practitioners Competence Assurance Act 2003: Report to the Minister of Health by the Director-General of Health*, Wellington, 2009, para. 2.1 and recommendation 2.
34 <http://www.midwiferycouncil.health.nz>.
35 The healthcare analysis company Dr Foster has produced a highly publicised *Hospital Guide* since 1981, comparing United Kingdom hospitals using hospital standardised mortality ratios: N. Hawkes, 'The mysterious Dr Foster', *British Medical Journal*, vol. 339, 2009, pp. 1336–37.
36 I. Kennedy, *Learning from Bristol: The Report of the Public Inquiry into*

37 *children's heart surgery at the Bristol Royal Infirmary 1984–1995*, Bristol Royal Infirmary Inquiry: United Kingdom, 2001, p. 3.

37 As occurred when the *Dominion Post* applied successfully to the Ombudsmen in 2007 for an order that the Capital and Coast District Health Board release sentinel and serious event information.

38 The Ministry of Health accepts that the 'outcome of credentialling – the credentialled status of a practitioner – should be in the public domain', and that '[w]here a practitioner's specific clinical responsibilities are less than their regulatory authority's scope of practice specifies, the reasons for this must be made explicit in the public record': Ministry of Health, *The Credentialling Framework for New Zealand Health Professionals*, Wellington, 2010, pp. 9–10.

39 Health Practitioners Competence Assurance Act 2003, s. 53.

40 Ibid., s. 58(1)(e).

41 Ibid., s. 60(1).

42 Ministry of Health response to Official Information Act request, September 2011.

43 Official Information Act 1982, s. 5.

44 Code of Health and Disability Services Consumers' Rights, right 7(8).

45 <http://www.myhospitals.gov.au/>.

46 S. Duckett et al., 'An improvement focus in public reporting: The Queensland approach', *Medical Journal of Australia*, vol. 189, 2008, pp. 616–17.

47 The subtitle of this section is inspired by N. Tomes, 'The "Information Rx"', in D. Rothman and D. Blumenthal (eds), *Medical Professionalism in the New Information Age*, pp. 40–65.

48 B. Bridgewater and B. Keogh, 'Surgical "league tables"', *Heart*, vol. 94, 2008, pp. 936–42.

49 E. Hannan et al., 'Improving the outcomes of coronary artery bypass surgery in New York State', *Journal of the American Medical Association*, vol. 271, 1994, pp. 761–66.

50 B. Bridgewater et al., 'Has the publication of cardiac surgery outcome data been associated with changes in practice in northwest England: An analysis of 25 730 patients undergoing CABG surgery under 30 surgeons over eight years', *Heart*, vol. 93, 2007, pp. 744–48.

51 P. Shekelle et al., *Does public release of performance results improve quality of care? A Systematic Review*, The Health Foundation: London, 2008.

52 Quoted in Society for Cardiothoracic Surgery in Great Britain & Ireland, 'Cardiac surgeons call for greater transparency and access to information for NHS patients', SCTS media statement, 21 March 2011.

53 Quoted in S. Boseley, G. Zorlu and R. Evans, 'Huge disparity in NHS death rates revealed', *Guardian*, 13 June 2010.

54 S. Westaby, N. Archer and N. Wilson, 'Media attack', Letter to editor, *British Medical Journal*, vol. 335, 2007, p. 839.

55 '*Le mieux est l'ennemi du bien*', in the words of Voltaire, *La Bégueule*, 1772.

56 M. Marshall et al., 'Public reporting on quality in the United States and the United Kingdom, *Health Affairs*, vol. 22, 2003, pp. 134–48 at p. 143.

57 Society for Cardiothoracic Surgery in Great Britain & Ireland, *Maintaining Patients' Trust*, p. 39.

58 B. Bridgewater, 'Why doctors' outcomes should be published in the press', *British Medical Journal*, vol. 331, 2005, p. 1210.

59 The New Zealand Joint Registry, compiled by the New Zealand Orthopaedic Association (with some Ministry of Health funding support) annually since 1999, is one example. It achieves 90% compliance (i.e., data contribution) for all hospitals undertaking joint replacement surgery in New Zealand. But the data, for example, on percentage of revisions, is aggregated and does not allow comparison by hospital, let alone orthopaedic surgeon.

60 S. McDonald, L. Excell and B. Livingston (eds), *The Thirty Third*

Report – Australia and New Zealand Dialysis and Transplant Registry, Australia and New Zealand Dialysis and Transplant Registry: Adelaide, 2010.
61 Health sector leaders' forum, Wellington, 2002.
62 S. Boseley, G. Zorlu and R. Evans, 'Huge disparity in NHS death rates revealed'.
63 M. Marshall et al., *Dying to Know: Public release of information about quality of health care*, Nuffield Trust: London, 2000, p. 75.
64 Quoted in S. Boseley, 'Heart surgeons push for other specialists to reveal death data', *Guardian*, 21 March 2011.
65 D. Geldard, 'Foreword: A patient's view', in Society for Cardiothoracic Surgery in Great Britain & Ireland, *Maintaining Patients' Trust*, p. 6.
66 Editorial, 'Public reporting of surgical outcomes', *Lancet*, vol. 377, 2011, p. 1126.
67 J. Semmens et al., 'The Western Australian Audit of Surgical Mortality: advancing surgical accountability', *Medical Journal of Australia*, vol. 183, 2005, pp. 504–8.
68 Royal Australasian College of Surgeons, *Australian and New Zealand Audit of Surgical Mortality – National Report 2009*, Adelaide, 2010.
69 Ibid., p. 3. A start has been made with the publication of Health Quality & Safety Commission, *Perioperative Mortality in New Zealand: Inaugural report of the Perioperative Mortality Review Committee*, Wellington, 2012. This initial report aggregates perioperative mortality data for 2005–2009 for four classes of procedures, but does not enable comparisons between regions.
70 I attended the symposium along with Ministers, senior officials, and health policy experts from the listed countries. I later recounted the experience at a parliamentary select committee hearing: see Health Committee, *2006/07 Financial Review of the Health and Disability Commissioner*, New Zealand House of Representatives: Wellington, 2008, pp. 10–11.
71 Since February 2008, the Quality Improvement Committee, and its successor the Health Quality & Safety Commission, has released aggregate 'serious and sentinel event' information reported from all district health boards. The first release was prompted by Official Information Act requests by the media. Public disclosure of such information is useful in highlighting the type of serious adverse events occurring in public hospitals, but variations in district health board reporting, and some sensationalist media reporting, render the process of limited utility. The latest report is Health Quality & Safety Commission, *Making Our Hospitals Safer: Serious and sentinel events reported by district health boards in 2010/11*, Wellington, 2012.
72 Personal communication, 2009.
73 District Health Boards New Zealand, *PHO Performance Results by DHB Region to June 2010*, Wellington, 2010.
74 P. Crampton et al., 'What makes a good performance indicator? Devising primary care performance indicators for New Zealand', *New Zealand Medical Journal*, vol. 117, 2004, pp. 1–12.
75 I. Kennedy et al., *Improving the Quality of Care in General Practice*, The King's Fund: London, 2011, p. 42.
76 Ibid., p. 41.
77 R. Mason, 'Patients to give GP surgeries TripAdvisor-style ratings', *Telegraph*, 8 December 2011, available at <http://www.telegraph.co.uk/health/healthnews/8941710/Patients-to-give-GP-surgeries-TripAdvisor-style-ratings.html>.
78 D. Williams, 'More performance data to be released under new transparency guidelines', *Health Service Journal*, 2 June 2011, available at <http://www.hsj.co.uk/news/primary-care/more-performance-data-to-be-released-under-new-transparency-guidelines/5030478>.

article>; and D. Williams and D. West, 'Exclusive: government to publish GP performance scorecards in transparency push', *Health Service Journal*, 6 July 2011, available at <http://www.hsj.co.uk/news/primary-care/exclusive-government-to-publish-gp-performance-scorecards-in-transparency-push/5032188.article>.
79 The Commonwealth Fund, *2006 International Health Policy Survey of Primary Care Physicians*, New York, 2006.
80 See D. Roter et al., 'Can e-mail messages between patients and physicians be patient-centred?', *Health Communication*, vol. 23, 2008, pp. 80–86; Y. Zhou et al., 'Patient access to an electronic health record with secure messaging: Impact on primary care utilization', *American Journal of Managed Care*, vol. 13, 2007, pp. 418–24; and R. Gauld, 'Factors associated with e-mail and internet use for health information and communications among Australians and New Zealanders', *Social Science Computer Review*, vol. 29, 2011, pp. 161–71.
81 See 'Can you trust your doctor', aired on 3 October 2011, available at <http://www.channel4.com/programmes/dispatches/articles/can-you-trust-your-doctor-feature>.
82 A. Esmail, 'Understanding patient safety in general practice', 3 October 2011, available at <http://blogs.bmj.com/bmj/2011/10/03/aneez-esmail-understanding-patient-safety-in-general-practice/#more-11568>.
83 Dr Ranchhod was eventually found guilty of professional misconduct and suspended: *Re Dr Ratilal Magan Ranchhod*, New Zealand Health Practitioners Disciplinary Tribunal, decision no. 273/Med09/129P, 21 December 2009.
84 Comments made by John Adams, chairman of the Medical Council, during interview on 'Nine to Noon', Radio New Zealand, 15 March 2010.
85 Editorial, 'Medical Council failed in its primary role', *Dominion Post*, 13 March 2010.
86 I have focused on recertification of doctors. There is a growing literature on recertification of other health practitioners: see, for example, Health Professions Council, *Continuing Fitness to Practise – Towards an evidence-based approach to revalidation*, London, 2009. For an overview of regulation of competence in other high-risk industries, see L. Donaldson, *Good Doctors, Safer Patients: Proposals to strengthen the system to assure and improve the performance of doctors and to protect the safety of patients. A report by the Chief Medical Officer*, Department of Health: London, 2006, ch. 7, pp. 133–43.
87 Comments made at Annual General Meeting of the Bay of Plenty branch of the New Zealand Medical Association, Tauranga, July 2001.
88 Health Practitioners Competence Assurance Act 2003, ss. 15(1)(c), 29(1).
89 Ibid., s. 4(3).
90 Ibid., s. 41(1).
91 Ibid., s. 41(3).
92 The Health Practitioner National Regulation Law 2009, ss. 35(1)(a), 109(1)(a)(iii).
93 Medical Board of Australia, *Continuing Professional Development Registration Standard*, 2010.
94 Australian Medical Council Specialist Education Accreditation Committee, *Accreditation of Specialist Medical Education and Training and Professional Development Programs: Standards and procedures*, Australian Medical Council: Canberra, 2010, standard 9.
95 I need to declare my interest in the MyCPD programme, as a current community member of the board of the Royal Australasian College of Physicians.
96 Royal Australasian College of Physicians, *Continuing Professional Development: Guide to MyCPD*, Sydney, 2008, p. 6.

97 N. Jenkins et al., 'The Effectiveness of Continuing Professional Development Project', in General Medical Council, *Publication of Proceedings. International Revalidation Symposium: Contributing to the evidence base*, London, 2011, pp. 53–56.

98 Medical Council of New Zealand, *Recertification and Continuing Professional Development*, Wellington, 2011, p. 7.

99 D. Kjeldmand and I. Holmstrom, 'Balint groups as a means to increase job satisfaction and prevent burnout among general practitioners', *Annals of Family Medicine*, vol. 6, 2008, pp. 138–45.

100 S. Lillis, 'The educational value of peer groups from a general practitioner perspective', *Journal of Primary Health Care*, vol. 3, 2011, pp. 218–21.

101 Medical Council of New Zealand, *Recertification and Continuing Professional Development*, p. 6.

102 R. Burgess, 'Clinical Audit and Revalidation', in *Publication of Proceedings. International Revalidation Symposium*, pp. 68–70.

103 The Medical Council of New Zealand has recognised the need to tighten the criteria for 'clinical audit', and in September 2011 issued a discussion paper for consultation.

104 I. Scott, G. Phelps and C. Brand, 'Assessing individual clinical performance: a primer for physicians', *Internal Medicine Journal*, vol. 41, 2011, pp. 144–55.

105 I. St George, 'PACman and Mrs MOPS – a challenge to educational orthodoxy', *New Zealand Family Physician*, vol. 28, 2001, pp. 310–12 at p. 310.

106 Ibid., p. 311 [emphasis in original].

107 Health and Disability Commissioner, *The Palms Medical Centre, Case 08HDC06359*, 30 June 2009, available at <http://www.hdc.org.nz/media/14106/08hdc06359medicalcentre.pdf>.

108 Health and Disability Commissioner, *Southland District Health Board Mental Health Services February–March 2001*, Auckland, 2002.

109 I. St George, 'Should all general practitioners be vocationally registered?', *New Zealand Family Physician*, vol. 31, 2004, pp. 17–19.

110 Ministry of Health, *The Credentialling Framework for New Zealand Health Professionals*, Wellington, 2010.

111 Health and Disability Commissioner, *The Palms Medical Centre, Case 08HDC06359*, p. 20.

112 J. Campbell, 'General registration – time for change', *New Zealand Doctor*, 4 June 2008, p. 20.

113 Ibid.

114 Medical Council of New Zealand media statement, 'Recertification: A new way forward', 16 December 2011.

115 Medical Council of New Zealand, *Recertification and Continuing Professional Development*, pp. 32–33.

116 Personal communication, October 2010.

117 Personal communication, senior staff at another Canadian college, October 2010.

118 The College of Family Physicians of Canada and the Royal College of Physicians and Surgeons of Canada.

119 W. Dauphinee, 'Self regulation must be made to work', *British Medical Journal*, vol. 330, 2005, pp. 1385–87.

120 G. Norman et al., 'Competency assessment of primary care physicians as part of a peer review program', *Journal of the American Medical Association*, vol. 270, 1993, pp. 1046–51 at p. 1046.

121 F. Goulet et al., 'Performance assessment. Family physicians in Montreal meet the mark!', *Canadian Family Physician*, vol. 48, 2002, pp. 1337–44.

122 N. Choudhry, R. Fletcher and S. Soumerai, 'Systematic review: The relationship between clinical experience and quality of health care', *Annals of Internal Medicine*, vol. 142, 2005, pp. 260–73.

123 College of Physicians and Surgeons of Ontario, *Annual Report 2010*, Toronto, 2011, p. 13; and personal communication,

124 Director, Quality Management Division, Ontario College, December 2011.
125 Personal communication, Registrar, Ontario College, November 2011.
126 W. Hall et al., 'Assessment of physician performance in Alberta: The Physician Achievement Review', *Canadian Medical Association Journal*, vol. 161, 1999, pp. 52–57.
127 W. Levinson, 'Revalidation of physicians in Canada: Are we passing the test?', *Canadian Medical Association Journal*, vol. 179, 2008, pp. 979–80.
128 New Zealand Medical Association chair Ross Boswell, quoted in K. Hayman, 'Patients fail in doctor diagnosis', *Dominion Post*, 7 February 2007.
129 K. Hayman, 'Patients fail in doctor diagnosis'.
130 W. Levinson, 'Revalidation of physicians in Canada', p. 980.
131 As was evident in letters to the *Canadian Medical Association Journal* in response to Levinson's editorial: *Canadian Medical Association Journal*, vol. 180, 2009, pp. 539–41.
132 T. Theman, H. Oetter and D. Kendel, 'Revalidation of Canadian physicians', *Canadian Medical Association Journal*, vol. 180, 2009, p. 539.
133 H. Chaudhry et al., 'Maintenance of licensure: Protecting the public, promoting quality health care', *Journal of Medical Regulation*, vol. 96, 2010, pp. 13–20.
134 S. Horowitz, S. Miller and P. Miles, 'Board certification and physician quality', *Medical Education*, vol. 38, 2004, pp. 10–11.
135 W. Levinson and M. Holmboe, 'Maintenance of certification in internal medicine', *Archives of Internal Medicine*, vol. 171, 2011, pp. 174–76.
136 N. Choudhry, R. Fletcher and S. Soumerai, 'Systematic review: the relationship between clinical experience and quality of health care'.
137 D. Davis et al., 'Accuracy of physician self-assessment compared with observed measures of competence: A systematic review', *Journal of the American Medical Association*, vol. 296, 2006, pp. 1094–102.
138 A. Audet et al., 'Measure, learn, and improve: Physicians' involvement in quality improvement', *Health Affairs*, vol. 24, 2005, pp. 843–53.
139 E. Holmboe, 'Assessment of the practicing physician: Challenges and opportunities', *Journal of Continuing Education in the Health Professions*, vol. 28, suppl. 1, 2008, pp. S4–S10.
140 See the lively debate in the *New England Medical Journal* where a striking majority (63%) of 2514 votes (with 80% cast by board-certified doctors) recommended *not* to enrol in the current ABIM MOC programme: P. Kritek and J. Drazen, 'American Board of Internal Medicine Maintenance of Certification Program – Polling Results', *New England Medical Journal*, vol. 362, 2010, pp. 948–52.
141 T. Brennan et al., 'The role of Physician Specialty Board certification status in the quality movement', *Journal of the American Medical Association*, vol. 292, 2004, pp. 1038–43.
142 The evidence is summarised in R. Lipner, 'The Role of Examinations in the Quality of Patient Care in the United States', in General Medical Council, *Publication of Proceedings. International Revalidation Symposium*, pp. 58–66.
143 E. Holmboe, 'Assessment of the practicing physician: Challenges and opportunities', pp. S4–S10.
144 Medical Act 1983, s. 29A(5).
145 J. Smith, *The Shipman Inquiry*, The Stationery Office: Norwich, 2004, Fifth Report, ch. 26.
146 L. Donaldson, *Good Doctors, Safer Patients: Proposals to strengthen the system to assure and improve the performance of doctors and to protect the safety of patients. A report by the Chief Medical Officer*, Department of Health: London, 2006.

146 Secretary of State for Health, *Trust, Assurance and Safety – The Regulation of Health Professionals in the 21st Century*, The Stationery Office: London, 2007.
147 House of Commons Health Committee, *Revalidation of Doctors. Fourth Report of Session 2010–11*, The Stationery Office: London, 2011.
148 J. Campbell, 'Evaluating the evidence base for supporting information for revalidation: Colleague questionnaires', in General Medical Council, *Publication of Proceedings. International Revalidation Symposium*, pp. 43–44.
149 J. Campbell et al., 'Factors associated with variability in the assessment of UK doctors' professionalism: Analysis of survey results', *British Medical Journal*, 27 October 2011, available at <http://www.bmj.com/content/343/bmj.d6212>.
150 See, for example, General Medical Council, *Good Medical Practice*, London, 2006; and Medical Council of New Zealand, *Good Medical Practice: A guide for doctors*, Wellington, 2008.
151 Medical Council of New Zealand, *Medical Council of New Zealand Annual Report 2010*, Wellington, 2010, p. 12.
152 E. McLean, 'Call for closer monitoring of doctors', *Otago Daily Times*, 2 August 2011.
153 I. Dickinson et al., 'Guide to the assessment of competence and performance in practising surgeons', *Australian and New Zealand Journal of Surgery*, vol. 79, 2009, pp. 198–204.
154 This was confirmed in the MORI poll commissioned in England in 2005. 'When asked what aspects of their doctor's performance they would like to comment on, the top characteristic was their communication skills followed by whether they are up to date, how much they involve patients in treatment decisions and whether they show their patients dignity and respect': L. Donaldson, *Good Doctors, Safer Patients*, para. 5, p. 146.

155 H. Sheldon, D. Swain and L. Harriss, *The Patient Voice in Revalidation: A discourse analysis*, Picker Institute Europe: Oxford, 2011.
156 Medical Council of New Zealand, *Recertification and Continuing Professional Development*, appendix 1, pp. 32–33.
157 The Medical Council's plans, which are well advanced, build on successful voluntary practice review programmes introduced by some colleges, notably the Royal Australian and New Zealand College of Obstetricians and Gynaecologists.
158 Under the Health Practitioners Competence Assurance Act 2003, ss. 36, 37.
159 <http://www.gmc-uk.org/about/role.asp>.
160 GfK NOP Social Research, *Research into Fitness for Practise Referrals 2011*, General Medical Council: London, 2011.
161 Further changes to the governance of the General Medical Council may result from the Government's expressed view that 'the system of directly appointed chairs is working well for those regulatory bodies which already have them' (Department of Health, *Enabling Excellence: Autonomy and accountability for healthcare workers, social workers and social care workers*, The Stationery Office: London, 2011, para. 3.14, p. 15). See also the review in September 2011 by the Council for Healthcare Regulatory Excellence, recommending smaller, non-representative boards, available at <http://www.chre.org.uk/_img/pics/library/pdf_1320922005.pdf>.
162 General Medical Council, *The State of Medical Education and Practice in the UK*, London, 2011.
163 General Medical Council, *Raising and acting on concerns about patient safety*, London, 2012.
164 See, for example, A. Mostrous, 'Scandal of killer doctors allowed to stay in

NHS', *The Times*, 3 November 2011. *The Times* reported that data obtained under the Freedom of Information Act showed that the GMC wanted 102 doctors erased from the register in 2010, but that fitness to practise panels (usually made up of two lay members and a doctor) allowed 40 doctors to remain registered – including a surgeon featured in the article, alleged to have botched operations that seriously injured or killed more than 20 patients, but still working under supervision in a London hospital.

165 My focus here is on medical regulators, but the same principles are applicable to all health practitioner regulatory bodies.

166 K. Shaw et al., 'Shared medical regulation in a time of increasing calls for accountability and transparency', *Journal of the American Medical Association*, vol. 302, 2008, pp. 2008–14.

167 The case for addressing the 'missing link' in a medical regulator's accountability to Parliament is well made by Donald Irvine: see D. Irvine and F. Hafferty, 'Every patient should have a good doctor', in the Society for Cardiothoracic Surgery in Great Britain & Ireland, *Maintaining Patients' Trust*, pp. 64–76 at p. 73. The Health Select Committee of the House of Commons in the UK is subjecting the work of the GMC to real scrutiny, with two inquiry reports in 2011.

168 Moves in this direction are already afoot in New Zealand: Cabinet Social Policy Committee, Minute of Decision, 'Proposed changes to health regulatory authorities', SOC Min(11) 15/5, 2011, released under the Official Information Act 1982.

169 H. Cayton, *Right-Touch Regulation*, Council for Healthcare Regulatory Excellence: London, 2010.

170 M. Bismark, M. Spittal and D. Studdert, 'Prevalence and characteristics of complaint-prone doctors in private practice in Victoria', *Medical Journal of Australia*, vol. 195, 2011, pp. 25–28.

EPILOGUE

1 Telephone conversation with Fay Bishop, October 2011.

2 H. Cayton, *Right-Touch Regulation*, Council for Healthcare Regulatory Excellence: London, 2010.

3 G. Colquhoun, *Playing God*, Steele Roberts: Wellington, 2002, p. 73.

4 L. Donaldson, *Good Doctors, Safer Patients: Proposals to strengthen the system to assure and improve the performance of doctors and to protect the safety of patients. A report by the Chief Medical Officer*, Department of Health: London, 2006.

SELECT BIBLIOGRAPHY

Ameringer, C., *State Medical Boards and the Politics of Public Protection*, The Johns Hopkins University Press: Baltimore, 1999.
Berger, J., *A Fortunate Man: The story of a country doctor*, Vintage Books: USA, 1997.
Berlinger, N., *After Harm: Medical error and the ethics of forgiveness*, The Johns Hopkins University Press: Baltimore, 2005.
Bosk, C., *Forgive and Remember: Managing medical failure*, The University of Chicago Press: Chicago, 1979.
Breen, K. et al., *Good Medical Practice: Professionalism, ethics and law*, Cambridge University Press: Melbourne, 2010.
Cartwright, S., *The Report of the Committee of Inquiry into Allegations Concerning the Treatment of Cervical Cancer at National Women's Hospital and into Other Related Matters*, Government Printing Office: Auckland, 1988.
Cayton, H., *Right-Touch Regulation*, Council for Healthcare Regulatory Excellence: London, 2010.
Chamberlain, J., *Doctoring Medical Governance: Medical self-regulation in transition*, Nova Science Publishers: New York, 2009.
Chisholm, A., Cairncross, L. and Askham, J., *Setting Standards: The views of members of the public and doctors on the standards of care and practice they expect of doctors*, Picker Institute Europe: Oxford, 2006.
Clarke, S. and Oakley, J. (eds), *Informed Consent and Clinical Accountability: The ethics of report cards on surgeon performance*, Cambridge University Press: Cambridge, 2007.
Coulter, A., *The Autonomous Patient: Ending paternalism in medical care*, Nuffield Trust: London, 2002.
——, *Engaging Patients in Healthcare*, Open University Press: Maidenhead, 2011.
—— and Collins, A., *Making Shared Decision-Making a Reality: No decision about me without me*, The King's Fund: London, 2011.
Cox, J. et al. (eds), *Understanding Doctors' Performance*, Radcliffe Publishing: Oxford, 2006.
Cull, H., *Review of Processes Concerning Adverse Medical Events*, Ministry of Health: Wellington, 2001.
Davies, G., *Queensland Public Hospitals Commission of Inquiry Report 2005*, Queensland Health: Brisbane, 2005.
Donaldson, L., *Good Doctors, Safer Patients: Proposals to strengthen the system to assure and improve the performance of doctors and to protect the safety of patients. A report by the Chief Medical Officer*, Department of Health: London, 2006.
Duffy, A., Barrett, D. and Duggan, M., *Report of the Ministerial Inquiry into the Under-Reporting of Cervical Smear Abnormalities in the Gisborne Region*, Ministry of Health: Wellington, 2001.
Dunbar, J., Reddy, P. and May, S., *Deadly Healthcare*, Australian Academic Press: Queensland, 2011.
Freckelton, I. (ed.), *Regulating Health Practitioners*, The Federation Press: Sydney, 2005.
Freidson, E., *Profession of Medicine: A study of the sociology of applied knowledge*, The University of Chicago Press: Chicago, 1988.
Gawande, A., *Complications: A surgeon's notes on an imperfect science*, Profile Books: London, 2002.
General Medical Council, *Good Medical Practice*, London, 2006.

———, *Publication of Proceedings. International Revalidation Symposium: Contributing to the evidence base*, London, 2011.
———, *The State of Medical Education and Practice in the UK*, London, 2011.
Gerteis, M. et al. (eds), *Through the Patient's Eyes: Understanding and promoting patient-centered care*, Jossey-Bass: San Francisco, 1993.
Gibson, R. and Singh, J., *Wall of Silence: The untold story of the medical mistakes that kill and injure millions of Americans*, LifeLine Press: Washington DC, 2003.
Grad, F. and Marti, N., *Physicians' Licensure and Discipline: The legal and professional regulation of medical practice*, Oceana Publications: New York, 1979.
Groopman, J., *How Doctors Think*, Houghton Mifflin: Boston, 2007.
Harpwood, V., *Medicine, Malpractice and Misapprehensions*, Routledge-Cavendish: Abingdon, 2007.
House of Commons Health Committee, *Revalidation of Doctors. Fourth Report of Session 2010–11*, The Stationery Office: London, 2011.
Irvine, D., *The Doctor's Tale. Professionalism and Public Trust*, Radcliffe Medical Press: Abingdon, 2003.
Jonsen, A., *The New Medicine & the Old Ethics*, Harvard University Press: Cambridge, 1990.
Kaplan, R., *Medical Murder: Disturbing cases of doctors who kill*, Allen & Unwin: New South Wales, 2009.
Kellogg, K., *Challenging Operations. Medical Reform and Resistance in Surgery*, The University of Chicago Press: Chicago, 2011.
Kennedy, I., *The Unmasking of Medicine*, Granada Publishing: London, 1983.
———, *Learning from Bristol: The report of the public inquiry into children's heart surgery at the Bristol Royal Infirmary 1984–1995*, Bristol Royal Infirmary Inquiry: United Kingdom, 2001.
——— et al., *Improving the Quality of Care in General Practice*, The King's Fund: London, 2011.
Lens, P. and van der Wal, G. (eds), *Problem Doctors: A conspiracy of silence*, IOS Press: The Netherlands, 1997.
Lown, B., *The Lost Art of Healing: Practicing compassion in medicine*, Houghton Mifflin: Boston, 1996.
Manning, J. (ed) *The Cartwright Papers: Essays on the Cervical Cancer Inquiry 1987–88*, Bridget Williams Books: Wellington, 2009.
Marshall, M. et al., *Dying to Know: Public release of information about quality of health care*, Nuffield Trust: London, 2000.
Medical Council of New Zealand, *Good Medical Practice: A guide for doctors*, Wellington, 2008.
Millenson, M., *Demanding Medical Excellence: Doctors and accountability in the information age*, The University of Chicago Press: Chicago, 1997.
O'Neill, O., *A Question of Trust*, Cambridge University Press: Cambridge, 2002.
Pringle, M., *Revalidation of Doctors: The credibility challenge*, Nuffield Trust: London, 2005.
Robinson, J., *A Patient's Voice at the GMC: A lay member's view of the General Medical Council*, Health Rights: London, 1988.
Rodwin, M., *Medicine, Money, and Morals: Physicians' conflicts of interest*, Oxford University Press: New York, 1993.
Rosenthal, M., *The Incompetent Doctor: Behind closed doors*, Open University Press: Buckingham, 1995.
———, Mulcahy, L. and Lloyd-Bostock, S. (eds), *Medical Mishaps: Pieces of the puzzle*, Open University Press: Buckingham, 1999.
Rothman, D. and Blumenthal, D. (eds), *Medical Professionalism in the New Information Age*, Rutgers University Press: New Jersey, 2010.

SELECT BIBLIOGRAPHY

Royal College of Physicians, *Doctors in Society: Medical professionalism in a changing world*, Report of a working party of the Royal College of Physicians of London, London, 2005.
——, *Future physician: Changing doctors in changing times*, Report of a working party, London, 2010.
Salter, B., *The New Politics of Medicine*, Palgrave Macmillan: Hampshire, 2004.
Secretary of State for Health, *Trust, Assurance and Safety – The Regulation of Health Professionals in the 21st Century*, The Stationery Office: London, 2007.
Shekelle, P. et al., *Does Public Release of Performance Results Improve Quality of Care? A systematic review*, The Health Foundation: London, 2008.
Smith, J., *The Shipman Inquiry*, The Stationery Office: Norwich, 2004.
Society for Cardiothoracic Surgery in Great Britain & Ireland, *Maintaining Patients' Trust: Modern medical professionalism*, Dentrite Clinical Systems: Henley-on-Thames, 2011.
St George, I. (ed.), *Cole's Medical Practice in New Zealand 2011*, Medical Council of New Zealand: Wellington, 2011.
Stacey, M., *Regulating British Medicine: The General Medical Council*, John Wiley & Sons: Chichester, 1992.
Stewart, J., *Blind Eye: How the medical establishment let a doctor get away with murder*, Simon & Schuster: New York, 1999.
Tallis, R., *Hippocratic Oaths: Medicine and its discontents*, Atlantic Books: London, 2004.
Thomas, H., *Sick to Death: A manipulative surgeon and a healthy system in crisis – A disaster waiting to happen*, Allen & Unwin: New South Wales, 2007.
Veatch, R., *Patient, Heal Thyself: How the 'new medicine' puts the patient in charge*, Oxford University Press: New York, 2008.
Walshe, K., *Regulating Healthcare: A prescription for improvement?*, Open University Press: Berkshire, 2003.
Walton, M., *The Trouble with Medicine: Preserving the trust between patients and doctors*, Allen & Unwin: Sydney, 1998.
Whittle, B. and Richie, J., *Prescription for Murder: The true story of Dr Harold Frederick Shipman*, Sphere: London, 2000.

INDEX

Accident Compensation Corporation (ACC), 102, 103–105
Accident Compensation Scheme, 101
accountability, 4, 15, 51, 55, 59, 63, 75–77, 84, 116, 122, 132
Action against Medical Accidents (AvMA) (UK), 82
adverse events, 26, 27, 54–55, 58, 103
Affordable Care Act 2010 (US), 72
Alberta Physician Achievement Review (PAR) programme, 144, 147
American Board of Internal Medicine (ABIM), 108–109, 135, 144, 149
American Board of Medical Specialties, 149
American Medical Association, 66
Code of Medical Ethics, 14
Ameringer, Carl, 79
assault, 50
Association of Salaried Medical Specialists, 66
audits, clinical, 98, 140, 143, 149, 152, 154
Australian and New Zealand Dialysis and Transplant Registry, 129
Australian Commission on Safety and Quality in Health Care, 64
Australian Health Practitioner Regulation Agency, 159–60
Australian Medical Association, 66

Berger, John, 5
Berwick, Don, 16, 129
Bismark, Marie, 26, 27
Blair, Ross, 76
Blumenthal, David, 16
Bolam rule, 93–96
Bolitho qualification, 94
Bosk, Charles, 89
Bottrill, Michael, 34, 39–41, 56, 70
Bottrill Inquiry, *see* Gisborne Cervical Screening Inquiry
Breen, Kerry, 75
Breeze, Ian, 98
Brennan, Troy, 104

Bridgewater, Ben, 128, 130
Bristol Inquiry, 16, 65, 75, 86, 121, 127
Bristol Royal Infirmary, 16, 121
British Medical Association (BMA), 66, 74
Broyard, Anatole, 12
Bundaberg Base Hospital, 37–39, 90, 97, 124
Burton, Mark, 141–42

callous conduct, 56–58
Campbell, John, 143
Campo, Rafael, 12
Canadian Medical Association (CMA), 66
cardiac surgery, lessons from, 126–30
Care Quality Commission (CQC) (UK), 130
Cartwright, Judge Silvia, 48, 115
Cartwright Inquiry, 6, 42, 48–49, 88
Centers for Medicare & Medicaid Services, 72–73
Cervical Cancer Inquiry, *see* Cartwright Inquiry
cervical screening programme, *see* National Cervical Screening Programme
Chantler, Cyril, 111
CME, *see* continuing medical education
Code of Health and Disability Services Consumers' Rights 1996, xi, 8, 10–11, 20–21, 46, 48, 92
Collège des Médecins du Québec, 145
College of Physicians & Surgeons of Alberta, 79, 147
College of Physicians and Surgeons of Ontario, 120, 146
colleges, professional, xv, 65, 84, 126, 138, 148–49, 154
Commonwealth Fund, 131
communication, 8–11, 55, 58, 75, 109, 115, 134, 147
comparative information, 42–43, 70–73, 112–14, 119, 121, 123–24, 126–33
compassion, 11–14
compensation schemes, 54, 94, 101, 102, 103, 104, 114, 116–17

198

INDEX

competence, xii–xviii, xix, 3–6, 8, 13–15, 17, 20, 22, 30–31, 33–34, 36–41, 43–44, 51, 56, 57, 64, 65, 66, 68–69, 73, 75–85, 87, 89, 90, 92–93, 98–101, 105, 106, 108–109, 112, 114, 115, 117, 118, 121–22, 134–39, 141–61, 165
competence review process, xv, 64, 66, 121, 135, 143–61
consent, 9–10
Constitution of the National Health Service (UK), 11
Consumer Health Reports, 119
Consumers Health Forum (Australia), 68
continuing medical education (CME), xiv, 137, 138, 141, 154
continuing professional development (CPD), xiv, 136–41, 143, 145, 151, 152, 153, 154, 155, 156, 162
Continuing professional development registration standard (Australia), 137
Coulter, Angela, 2
Council for Healthcare Regulatory Excellence (CHRE) (UK), 157, 159, 160
courts, 64, 94, 97, 98, 99, 100
CPD, *see* continuing professional development
credentialling, xv, 38, 43, 121, 142, 156
Cull, Helen, 102–103
Cull Inquiry, 102–103, 104
culture, medical, 9, 11, 16, 36, 76, 83–93, 106, 110, 127

Davies, Geoffrey, 38
defensive medicine, 67, 76
disciplinary proceedings, 7, 8, 28, 43, 44, 45, 46, 51, 53, 55, 65, 66, 68, 79–80, 81, 86, 87, 102, 114–17, 120, 121, 125, 147
disciplinary tribunal, 42, 44, 46, 47, 53, 64–65, 100, 102, 116, 120
Doctors4Justice (UK), 82
Donaldson, Liam, 22, 150

employers, 38, 52, 55, 63, 71, 97, 98, 99, 101, 125
Esmail, Aneez, 134
expert advisors, 29, 87–88, 93–96, 100
exploitation,
  financial, 7, 45–47, 116
  sexual, 45–47, 116

Fahey, Morgan, 46

Federation of Medical Regulatory Authorities of Canada, 144
Federation of State Medical Boards (US), 120, 148
Federation of Women's Health Councils Aotearoa New Zealand, 4
Finnigan, Judge Daniel, 99
Freidson, Eliot, 15

Galgut, Damon, 2
Gawande, Atul, 32, 90
General Medical Council (GMC) (UK), 2, 9, 35, 36, 65, 68, 69, 77, 78, 79, 82, 109, 117, 133, 134, 150–51, 157–58
general practice/practitioners, 12, 28, 36, 62, 34–36, 44, 46, 53, 62, 77, 94, 112, 125, 131–33, 141–43
general registrants, 141–43
Gerada, Clare, 132
Gisborne Cervical Screening (Bottrill) Inquiry, 39–41
Gisborne Hospital, 48, 52–53
Green, Herbert, 6, 48

Harpwood, Vivienne, 74
Hasil, Roman, 58, 80
Haslam, Michael, 46
Health and Disability Commissioner (HDC), x, xi, 26, 27, 28, 29, 30, 31, 37, 42, 43, 49, 68, 87, 94, 95, 98–99, 100, 102, 103, 115, 118, 134, 142, 143, 159, 162–63
Health and Disability Commissioner Amendment Act 2003, 103
Health Practitioner Regulation National Law 2009, 92
Health Practitioners Competence Assurance Act 2003, 76, 103, 136, 153, 160
Health Select Committees, 64, 125, 133, 151, 157
Healthcare complaint commissions, 64, 100, 101, 159
Helman, Cecil, xvi
Herceptin, 70
hindsight bias, 96
Hippocratic Oath, 14, 84
Holloway, Linda, 88
Holmboe, Eric, 149, 150
House of Commons Health Committee (UK) 133, 151, 157, *see also* Health Select Committees

INDEX

ImPatient for Change (Canada), 69
indemnity insurers, 66, 101, 115, 116–17
information disclosure, 41–45, 70–73, 112–33
information silos, 101–105
informed consent, 42, 44, 45, 48–49, 71, 75, 113
inquiries, official, 34–42
Irvine, Donald, 2, 5, 17, 82, 83

Jonsen, Albert, 13, 14

Kennedy, Ian, 16, 86, 121
Keogh, Bruce, 127
Kerr, William, 46

Lansley, Andrew, 151
league tables, 128
legal constraints, 93–105
Levinson, Wendy, 8, 148

Maddern, Guy, 131
Maimonides, 13–14
Maintenance and Enhancement of Physician Performance, 145
Maintenance of Certification (MOC), 149
Maintenance of Licensure framework, 148
maintenance of professional standards (MOPS) programmes, 84, 138
managers, health, 63, 74, 91, 97
Manning, Joanna, 104, 116
Marshall, Martin, 9, 70–71, 111, 128
McIntyre, Neil, 87
McMullin, Sir Duncan, 51
Mechanic, David, 74
media, xv, 2, 4, 66–67, 75, 102, 121, 127, 128, 129, 133, 134, 135, 148, 158
Medical Act 1983 (UK), 150
Medical Board of Australia, 39, 117, 137, 138, 153
  Code of Conduct, 14
Medical Board of Queensland, 38
medical boards, *see* regulators, medical
Medical Council of New Zealand, 18, 30, 31, 37, 43, 47, 52–53, 57, 77, 80, 81, 89, 91–92, 103, 104, 105, 109, 110, 118, 119, 120, 121, 134–35, 136, 138, 139, 142, 143, 153, 154, 156, 166
Medical Law Reform Group, 51
medical manslaughter, 51–52
medical murder, xiii, 7, 34–35, 49–50

Medical Practitioners Disciplinary Tribunal, 102
Medical Professionalism in the New Millennium charter, 16–17
Medical Protection Society, 66, 118
Mello, Michelle, 117
Midwifery Council of New Zealand, 121
Millenson, Michael, 71–72
Ministry of Health (NZ), 119, 122, 131
morbidity and mortality meetings, 89–90
MyCPD programme, 138–39

National Cervical Screening Programme, 34, 40–41
National Health Service (NHS) (UK), 56, 72, 117, 127, 130, 132, 151
  NHS Litigation Authority (NHSLA), 101, 116, 117
National Practitioner Data Bank (US), 117, 120
National Women's Hospital, xi, 6, 48
Nationwide Health & Disability Consumer Advocacy Service, 11
natural justice, 96–99
negligent harm, 54–56
New Zealand Medical Association (NZMA), 66, 74, 88
New Zealand Medical Council, *see* Medical Council of New Zealand
Norman, Geoffrey, 145

ObamaCare reforms, 72
Ombudsmen, 43, 55, 64, 122
O'Neill, Onora, 71, 76–77
Osler, William, 2, 20
outcome bias, 96

Parry, Graham, 102
Patel, Jayant, 34, 37–39, 52, 70, 80, 90, 92, 97, 124
Patel Inquiry, *see* Queensland Inquiry
patient
  advocacy groups, xii, 3, 4, 51, 62, 68
  autonomy, 16, 19, 42, 47, 113
  expectations, 20–21, 26, 55, 67, 108, 109, 110, 156, 161
  exploitation, 7, 45–49, 116
  views, 3–13
Patients Association (UK), 68

INDEX

Paul, Charlotte, 88
Peabody, Francis, 13
peer review, 79, 83, 84, 136, 137, 138, 139–41, 143, 145, 146, 147, 148, 154
Performance Achievement Review (PAR), 147–48
Peters, James, 50
Pharmac, 70
Picker Institute, 5, 68
Pilot Performance Evaluation Programme, 148
Pizzo, Philip, 8
policy-makers, xv, 63–64, 70, 72, 84, 101
Popper, Karl, 87
Poutsma, Colleen, 102
Practice Improvement Modules (PIMs), 149
primary health organisations (PHOs), 131–32

quality assurance/improvement, xvii, xviii, 18, 20, 34, 38–39, 41–43, 62, 63, 64, 72, 77, 79, 83, 84, 94, 96, 99, 101, 108–109, 110, 112–14, 119, 122–33, 136, 141, 144, 145–60
Quality Outcomes Framework (UK), 77
Queensland (Patel) Inquiry, 37–39, 80
Queensland Health, 38–39, 124
Queensland Public Hospitals Commission of Inquiry Report, 38–39

Ranchhod, Ratilal, 134
recertification, xv, 15, 34, 36, 37, 70, 77, 108, 111, 112, 133, 135–38, 140, 141, 142, 144–60
reckless harm, 52–53
Reeves, Graeme, 50, 92
regulators, medical, xv, 18, 55, 59, 65, 78–83, 91, 92, 106, 108, 109, 110, 117, 118, 120, 121, 125, 135, 136, 142, 145, 146, 148, 150, 152, 153–60
rehabilitation, doctor, 52, 79, 81
Resident Doctors' Association, 66
revalidation, *see* recertification
review of practice, scope, 100–101
Robinson, Jean, 69, 83–84
Rosenthal, Marilynn, 33, 90–91
Royal Australasian College of Pathologists, 39, 41
Royal Australasian College of Physicians, 138, 154

Royal Australasian College of Surgeons, 130–31, 154
Royal College of General Practitioners, 132

Sassall, John, 13
sexual misconduct, 7, 46
Shipman, Harold, xiii, 34–37, 49, 70
Shipman Inquiry, xiii, 34–37, 39, 65, 69, 75, 77, 89, 133, 134, 150
Shirkey, Kay, 141, 143
Simiao, Sun, 13
Smith, Dame Janet, xiii, 34, 36, 69, 82, 89, 133, 150
Smith, Richard, 32, 75
Society for Cardiothoracic Surgery of Great Britain & Ireland (SCTS), 126–27, 130
Southland Hospital, 142
specialty boards, *see* colleges, professional
St George, Ian, 141
Stacey, Margaret, 78
Studdert, David, 104
surgeons, 6, 34, 37–39, 49, 51, 57, 72, 89–90, 92, 97, 98, 101, 108, 121, 126–31
Swango, Michael, 49–50

Taggart, David, 127
Tallis, Raymond, 71, 75, 83
Tauranga Hospitals Inquiry, 80, 98, 100
Tomes, Nancy, 114

United Kingdom Department of Health, 130, 132

Veatch, Robert, 19
vocational registration, 28, 43, 65, 141–43, 156

Walsh, Peter, 82
Wanganui Hospital, 58, 80
Wellington Hospital, 87–88
Whanganui District Health Board Inquiry, 99
whistle-blowers, 37, 85, 101
Women's Health Action, 68